How to Give Yourself

Relief from Pain

by the Simple Pressure of a Finger

Dr. Roger Dalet

STEIN AND DAY/*Publishers*/New York

First published in the United States of America in 1980.
Copyright © 1978 by Opera Mundi
Translation © 1980 by Stein and Day, Inc.
All rights reserved.
Printed in the United States of America
Stein and Day/*Publishers*/Scarborough House,
Briarcliff Manor, N.Y. 10510

Library of Congress Cataloging in Publication Data

Dalet, Roger.
  How to give yourself relief from pain by the simple pressure of a finger.

  Translation of Supprimez vous-même vos douleurs par simple pression d'un doigt.
  1. Acupressure. I. Title.
RM723.A27D3513   1980   615.8'22   79–3825
ISBN 0–8128–2711–2

Photographs by M. Conty

Contents

Sexuality

The Scientific Explanation

Introduction

Although we traditionally speak only of five senses — touch, taste, smell, hearing, and sight — there is a sixth sensation that is the most severe and disturbing and that demands attention and relief: *pain*. While most of us would regard pain as totally evil, it is also, paradoxically, an important survival mechanism as those very few people who are born without the ability to perceive pain know to their chagrin. They continually suffer injury in circumstances where the rest of us would have received warning signals.

While pain has a value by calling our attention to something that is wrong and that may need medical attention, that is no reason to live with it once it has achieved its purpose. Pain often, if not usually, has disadvantages that far outweigh its benefits. Sometimes the warning pain turns out to be a false alarm; or the signal may give a disproportionately exaggerated indication of the underlying cause, which may be trivial. Such pain may be disabling while serving no purpose, and it is pain such as this that we are aiming to treat in this book.

Everyone these days has heard of acupuncture. Until recently most of us tended to think of it as a secret, very mysterious, and very complicated oriental method of medical treatment. But with the opening up of China to foreign visitors, many reports have emerged of major surgical operations being performed under acupuncture anesthesia alone and of the use of acupuncture to treat a wide variety of conditions — even some, such as deafness, that are not particularly associated with pain. Films of this treatment have been shown on television, and reports have been published in the serious scientific medical journals of Europe and America.

In China itself, thousands of men and women, the so-called "barefoot doctors," have been trained to look after, relieve, or cure the complaints and ailments of their own families, their neighbors, and their fellow workers, and to do this simply by stimulating certain selected points on the body.

Anyone can learn to relieve his own aches and pains, and those of his children, friends, and neighbors, by the same methods. We are not talking here about the full system of acupuncture treatment. This is the province of the professional acupuncturists. We are talking, rather, about a method of obtaining quick, even if sometimes only temporary, relief: a method simpler to apply, but based on exactly the same principles as acupuncture; a method, which is at least as effective as taking pills or other medicine, for the relief of such complaints as backache, colds, headache, and many other troublesome aches. This method can also be used to cure some complaints that are not especially painful but are disturbing, such as insomnia.

Historical Background

Traditional methods of treatment in Chinese medicine, whether using needles or the application of heat, go back to the beginning of time.

Recent excavation of prehistoric tombs has turned up more and more often needles that were undoubtedly used for therapeutic purposes. Often these needles are simply splinters chipped from small pointed stones or flints, but gold and silver needles, somewhat oxidized over the years, have been found in the tombs of nobles and kings.

There are very few original documents relating to the origins of the ancient science of acupuncture, and there is therefore an abundance of hypotheses about the beginnings of this practice; there are even people who think that the origin and growth of this method of medicine, so peculiar to China, may be explained by a visit from outer space. But without going quite so far, one can—we think—willingly accept that the reports of scrupulously careful and critical observers from the West, at the invitation of the Chinese, have allowed this whole important structure, which for us is a new, and, on the surface of it, strange system of medicine, to be brought to Western consciousness.

Early in the history of China, people tried to systematize the practice of acupuncture. As early as 220 B.C., an important work called the *Nei-*

King, Nei-Jing, or *Nei-Ching,* was commissioned by the Emperor Houang-Ti, the "Yellow Emperor." He wrote in one of his edicts, "I am disturbed by the amount in taxes and dues that do not reach me on account of illness among the people. My wish is that we should no longer use medicine, which poisons them, or ancient methods. I want those mysterious metal needles, which direct energy, to be used instead."

The whole of acupuncture rests on this phrase, and over the succeeding centuries, careful, patient, and repeated observations have allowed the method in all its aspects to be defined.

The practice flourished and was widely used and taught. Around A.D. 1400 the bronze statuette known as the bronze man, a statue pierced with holes corresponding to the acupuncture points on the skin, was being used as a model to teach students.

The use of acupuncture suffered an eclipse toward the beginning of the nineteenth century when invading Europeans influenced the élites of Chinese society to introduce the methods of Western medicine. In particular, during the last years of the government that preceded the present regime in China, traditional medicine was outlawed and was able to survive only in remote country areas. It was not until Mao Tse-tung came to power that traditional medicine was generally reinstated and came to be both practiced and taught in hospitals as well as in workplaces where "barefoot doctors" could treat their fellow workers. Today medical research and therapeutics in China are more or less split between traditional and Western methods, as Mao Tse-tung had wished.

The underlying theory of acupuncture is complex, but the main principles are clearly defined. Here we shall describe them and use them as a skeleton for as much additional theory as is necessary.

Above all, acupuncture is a philosophy, or rather a method of treatment, that has been incorporated into the Chinese cosmological and philosophical tradition. In classical Chinese thought, the world of matter and the world of energy are a continuity. We can draw a striking parallel between this binary system and that defined in the West by Einstein and his followers.

In the Chinese tradition, the two elements of this binary system are called Yin and Yang; they symbolize the light and dark aspects of things, and these two forces completely complement each other and merge into one another without disturbing each other as inevitably as day follows night and ice becomes water. They are, in short, two aspects or sides of the same truth.

This binary system underlies the whole structure and functioning of matter, and matter, according to the Chinese, is composed of five different elements. (Numbers were very important in ancient Chinese philosophy—after all, it was they who, through the Persians and the

Arabs, gave us our present system of numbers—and the number five was particularly significant to them.)

So there are five cardinal points (the Chinese add the center to the four that we describe), five planets, five tastes, five smells; and there are also five elements—earth, fire, water, air, and wood; and each of these five elements are held to correspond with one of our specific organs. And all of this intermingles, through a network of correspondences. It is as if the ancient Chinese philosophers had predicted the French poet Baudelaire's famous phrase: *"Les parfums, les couleurs, et les sons se répondent."**

But it is also interesting that ancient Greek medicine—and indeed Western medicine until relatively modern times—was based on the very similar system of the four elements: earth, air, fire, and water; the four properties: hot, cold, wet, and dry; and the four humors: blood, phlegm, yellow bile, and black bile. The humors were believed to correspond not only to the appropriate mixture of these elements and properties but also to the seasons of the year and the temperaments and dispositions of individual people. So there was, in earlier times, a link between the foundations on which Chinese and Western medical theory rested.

But acupuncture is not only a philosophical theory; it is also a system of medicine and a technique of treatment. It is always interesting to see the different ways in which traditional Chinese doctors work in the operating theater as compared with Western doctors. Like the Western doctor, the Chinese doctor makes a diagnosis; but to do this, he uses elements that are disregarded by Western doctors. He examines carefully the patient's face, his expression, the color of his eyes, the color and grain of his skin; he examines, quite literally millimeter by millimeter, the patient's tongue; and in so doing he discovers the correspondences with the central organs. He feels the abdomen, but not in the way that a Western doctor does, looking for the size of the liver, spleen, and other organs, but very lightly and gently, stroking almost, each region of the abdominal wall. This tells him things about the workings of the organs and about the person in general. And finally, above all, he takes the pulse.

In the West, we consider that we have only one pulse, although it may be felt in many of our arteries. In China, it is thought that there are twelve pulses, corresponding to the organs, which are palpated with extreme sensitivity of touch, an extraordinary skill from which the acupuncturist gains a wealth of knowledge.

* The smells, colors, and sounds commune with one another."—from Baudelaire's sonnet *"Correspondences"* in the *Fleurs du Mal*.

The Chinese doctor then moves on to therapy. The important thing to understand about the application of his therapeutic rules is that according to the Chinese conception, vital energy flows constantly throughout the body; in health this energy is made up of a balanced mixture of Yin and Yang. There is a continuous flow of this vital energy both over the entire surface of the body and along the special lines of channels that correspond with the major organs. There is thus a line, which we in the West call a meridian, that corresponds with the heart, another with the lungs, another with the liver, and others with the spleen, the kidneys, the small and large intestines, the bile ducts, the bladder, and the stomach. There are other meridians that correspond to other functions. Finally, there are supplementary or connecting meridians that link all the main vessels together into a complex network.

If energy stops flowing, in other words if there is an obstruction somewhere along one of these meridians or if there is an imbalance of the proportions of the Yin and the Yang, illness will develop. In the same way, from a qualitative point of view, if a perverse energy replaces the normal vital energy, illness will result. Now along these meridians there are points—361 in all, plus a few scattered separate ones—that allow the flow of energy to be modified both qualitatively and quantitatively. And once the doctor is well informed about the patient through his initial examination, he is able, according to complex rules, called by poetic names such as Mother-Son Rule or Rule of the Five Elements, to place small needles in carefully and specifically chosen spots so that the normal flow of qualitatively correct energy may reestablish itself, and, as a result, good health will return.

When such theories were introduced in the West, they provoked shock and outrage since they failed completely to correspond with any established anatomical or physiological observations; after all, no one has actually observed these meridians; and for this reason, on the various occasions when Chinese medicine was introduced and reintroduced into the West, it soon fell into disrepute and was finally abandoned, until very recently that is. In the sixteenth century the Benedictines, returning from China, first expounded the fundamentals of Chinese medicine and brought back acupuncture needles; but they only aroused sarcasm. Then, during the nineteenth century, a number of doctors, including the father of the composer Berlioz, wrote about the advantages of the strange technique. But among the successes there were also failures and accidents, and again the method was quickly disregarded and the theory dismissed. Not until the end of the nineteenth century, when lay observers—not doctors—such as Soulié de Morant, who was a French consul in China and who studied Chinese medicine and translated Chinese texts, did the practice again begin to spread in the West.

The most recent introduction has occurred during the last few years, but even today acupuncture arouses scepticism, and even hostility, among many Western therapists and research scientists.

But alongside the doubters, there are those who have tried acupuncture and whose successful results have fired them with enthusiasm. So we may say that the debate is still going on in the West, even though it has no real reason to since traditional acupuncture has undergone considerable development and change, above all in its country of origin.

We have seen that in modern China, under Mao Tse-tung, it was felt to be important to build a bridge between modern Western science and the traditional Chinese approach. Chinese doctors have adopted Western methods and adapted them where necessary to complement their own (and Western doctors have been amazed by the results). This association of techniques has taken place principally in the area of general care and hygiene in clinics and hospitals. Westerners visiting China have been particularly astonished to find surgery, without conventional anesthesia, being performed on a patient where analgesia, that is to say absence of pain, is achieved simply by inserting a needle into a specific point in the body. Patients have been filmed and interviewed during the course of their operations — people who, for example, were having a lung or part of the stomach removed, or mothers who were giving birth by Caesarian section, while still awake and fully conscious. This was something that was totally unbelievable until we were given visual proof.

This system of medicine has been taught right down to the level of the barefoot doctors; even factory workers and farm laborers have learned how to use the needles and thus relieve the afflictions of their fellow workers, neighbors, and family. Some of the barefoot doctors have even been encouraged to conduct their own research; one of them, Tchao Pou Yu, has become a popular hero because of his success in treating the deaf and dumb.

Chinese doctors and scientists have also greatly improved on their acupuncture techniques. They have discovered effective new points; they have discovered new paths that complement the known existing ones and that link up skin points to the major organs; and they have experimented with new methods, in particular with sending an electric current through the acupuncture needles. Above all, the contemporary Chinese have greatly simplified the use of acupuncture, through repeated experimentation during treatment and surgery; in particular, they have considerably reduced the number of points used for treating different complaints. Often one point alone is enough to cover an entire region, whatever the pathological condition. Safe and effective treatment can now be given in the simplest of ways. And recent exciting discoveries made by Western scientists at last provide a scientific basis, acceptable to the Western tradition, for the use of acupuncture. These are described in the last section of this book.

In any event, whatever the way in which acupuncture works, by using all the knowledge now available, we can, if not cure ourselves completely, at least relieve our complaints by the application of pressure to a small number of specific points on the body.

In this book we are going to look at and describe the stimulation of these pressure points.

How to Use This Book

Acupuncture points have been well known in China from earliest times, and most of them are held to correspond to specific organs and areas of the body. Acupuncturists work by inserting needles of varying lengths at these points. When they are stimulated, the corresponding area is being treated and responds to the stimulation.

How do you apply the stimulation? First, carefully locate the points, as described in the following pages: each point occupies only a very small area, approximately half a square millimeter. The diagrams and explanations that follow will enable you to locate them easily. Once they are located, you cannot mistake them since they are highly sensitive areas and the feeling is quite different from the surrounding tissues. There is a scientific reason for this as will be described later.

Having located the points, you now have to stimulate them. The acupuncturist will, of course, insert his needle, but pressing on the point can be almost as effective.

Place the tip of your index or second finger or thumb on the point, and press down forcefully, vibrating your finger slightly, giving a rapid little massage, while rotating your finger clockwise.

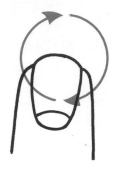

If you want to be even more precisely on the point, you can use a small object such as a pencil eraser or the end of a ballpoint pen. You can even adapt a thimble by glueing to its end a small rounded tip of a size that just covers the exact area. The thimble end may also be warmed to apply heat, but use it carefully. This little device may be found very effective, as may other small instruments such as electric vibrators; but the simplest instrument of all is the tip of the finger.

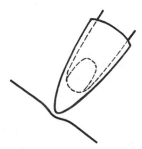

The length of time for which relief lasts will vary from patient to patient, from a few minutes to several hours or even days, but the effectiveness of the point will not vary through use, and the same result will be obtained time and time again.

It is, of course, usually more difficult to notice a result when the complaint is less painful, but the principle is always the same, however serious the ailment—continue stimulating the point until you feel relief.

Let us now look at certain common complaints and the tiny acupressure points that are the key to relieving them.

The chapters are arranged according to the part of the body affected.

The Head and Neck

Relief for an Earache

Surprising though it may seem, there are really three ears — or, at least, three parts that lead into one another: the external ear, that is, the outer shell and the auditory canal that leads to the drum; the middle ear, a resonating cavity with four linked small bones that transmit the sound; and the inner ear, which registers the sounds and, among other things, contains the mechanism that enables us to keep our balance. The inner ear does not give us pain — disturbance in it is manifested in other ways, such as dizziness, ringing in the ears, deafness, and so on, and we are not concerned with that here.

In contrast, the other two parts of the ear may become painful. Small boils can develop on the outer ear, and they can be very painful. More seriously, there can be infection in the middle ear — which becomes the seat of what is medically known as otitis, which is extremely painful and may lead to complications, particularly in the neighboring bone, the mastoid. Complications usually mean partial loss of hearing, which (especially before antibiotics were available) sometimes affects the patient for the rest of his life. Small children are particularly vulnerable to ear infection.

There is a point that will relieve
simple earache. It is located just
behind the ear on the mastoid bone.
Pull the ear forward, and the point is
just on the bone.

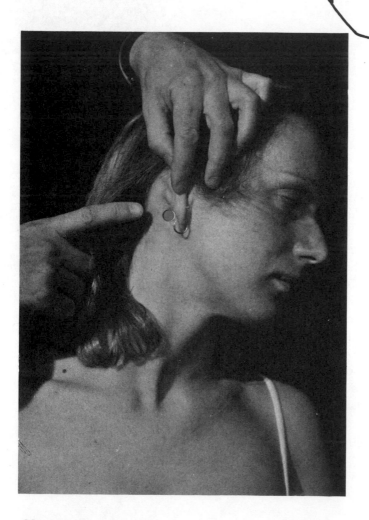

Relief for Aching Eyes

Your eyes may feel painful for a number of reasons: a blow, a speck of dust, or an infection such as conjunctivitis. There are also more serious causes, such as iritis or glaucoma, to mention the major ones that endanger the vision. To protect your eyesight, consult a doctor as soon as possible if your eyes start to ache. He will conduct a careful examination of the eyes, in particular the back of the eye, the retina, and the nerve that collects the visual images and transmits them to the brain. He will also measure the tension in the eye. Hypertension indicates glaucoma, which can destroy vision within hours.

In the meantime we suffer and perhaps can scarcely see since the other eye may also shut protectively as a reflex.

There is one point that can bring rapid relief.

This point is located close to the healthy eye, near the inside corner.

Press on the left point firmly to treat the right eye, and vice versa. If both eyes are inflamed, use both points simultaneously.

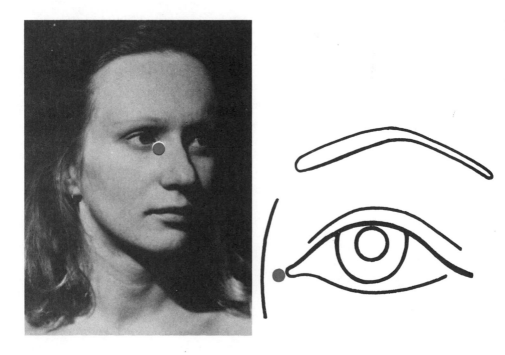

A Tonic for the Facial Muscles

Women have always been criticized for spending hours in front of a mirror. Yet some people argue that beauty is a gift that ought to be cared for. While the surface of the body depends on the quality of its foundations, there are virtually no prescribed methods of maintaining the facial muscles. While we maintain our biceps and exercise our abdominal muscles, we neglect our many tiny facial muscles — those, as Darwin wrote, that express our emotions, our laughter, and smiles, but which, when relaxed, betray our wrinkles and reveal our sagging, aging features.

So acupuncture finds its place in beauty care. Regular stimulation of points on the face tones up muscles and delays the appearance of aging.

There are several points on the face. We have chosen six, three on each side.

The first is on the forehead, two finger-widths beyond the outer end of the eyebrow and four finger widths above it. The second is on the underside of the cheekbone, facing the nose. The third is located exactly at the corner of the mouth, one finger-width away from where the lips meet.

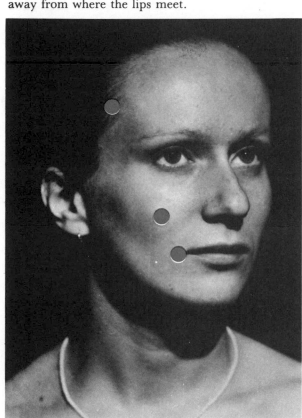

Controlling Facial Pain

Pains in the face are among the least endurable, whether the patient is suffering from facial neuralgia or less easily diagnosed conditions.

Facial neuralgia is a quite specific pain. It is common in older people and occurs quite suddenly after grazing or stimulating a susceptible area on the cheek, the nose, or the gums. This area is almost always the same for each patient and is called the trigger zone. The pain is typical: it occurs in a flash, like an electric shock, lasting only a few seconds; but, so the patient tells us, what seconds! The pain is agonizing and makes the sufferer's life a misery.

In contrast to this quite specific pain, there are several varieties of a different sort of discomfort, where the pain is less intense but more persistent. Often the face becomes red and the patient sweats. The condition is very unpleasant, and it is useful to know some points that can bring relief.

There are several points, but two main ones. The first, which is suitable for migraines and other headaches as well as facial pains, is located on the inside of the forearm — use the opposite arm to the side of the pain.

Grip with the thumb and index finger around the thumb of the other hand, and the index finger will point to the exact spot.

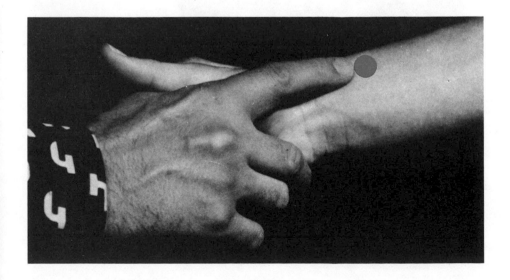

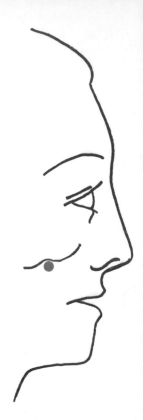

The second point is located on the face, level with the nostril in the bony groove under the cheek.

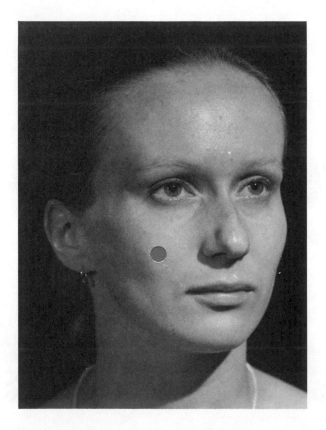

To Prevent Fainting

Fainting and loss of consciousness may be caused by a number of things. Some are serious. You may feel faint after sudden and intense physical pain, such as severe renal colic or a coronary thrombosis. But in the majority of cases, the situation, while dramatic, is less serious. You may, for example, feel faint after hearing bad news, or again if you have low blood pressure you are likely to feel faint when suddenly sitting or standing up after lying down for some time. Or you may be one of those people who have a tendency to fainting attacks because of slowing of the heart rate.

Whatever the cause, in such a situation you need to act quickly.

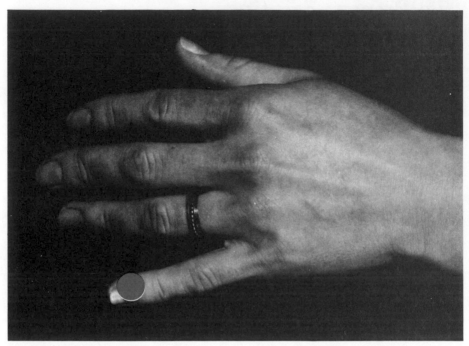

The two points effective for overcoming faintness are on the little finger on the ring finger side, at the right angle formed by a line along the base of the fingernail with a vertical line down the side of the nail. You will need to lay the patient down and press forcefully.

If you are applying the pressure to yourself, you can do this lying down, using your folded thumb.

Forceful pressure revives the patient and prevents the loss of consciousness.

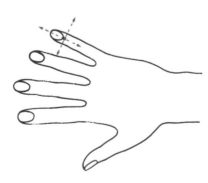

Relief for a Headache

Headaches are perhaps more common than aches in any other part of the body. There are a large number of causes, from flu to indigestion to a brain tumor, not to mention eyestrain or any number of psychosomatic causes.

A careful medical examination is necessary to diagnose the real trouble, but in the meantime relief can be provided by one of three points, depending on the exact site of the headache.

1. Headache on the forehead or temples, on one or both sides.
2. Headache on the nape of the neck and back of the head.
3. Headache in the skull and generally all over.

1. For headache on the forehead or temples, on one or both sides, the effective point is located on the wrist, where the pulse is taken, but a little higher toward the elbow. To locate it accurately, on the right wrist for example, hold your right hand flat, palm upward and thumb out. Lock your right thumb over your left hand thumb, and with the three smaller fingers on your left hand wrapped around your right hand. You will find that your index finger held straight will point exactly to the point.

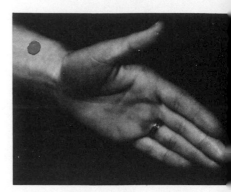

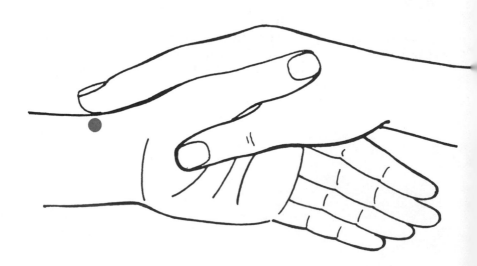

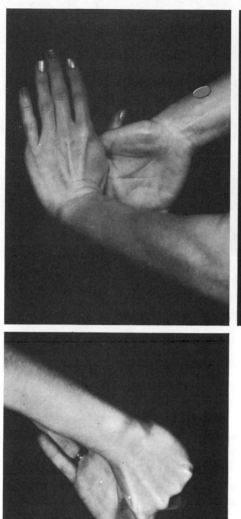

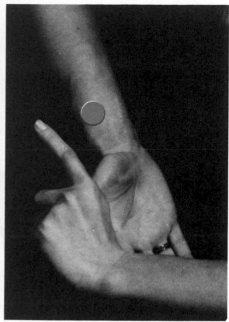

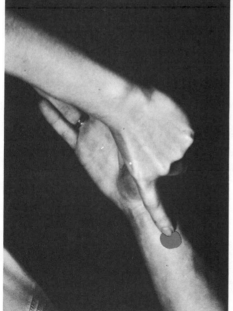

If your entire forehead aches, you should stimulate the point on both wrists. If only one side hurts, stimulate the point on the opposite wrist; that is, if the headache is on the right side, stimulate the left wrist; for a headache on the left side, use the right wrist.

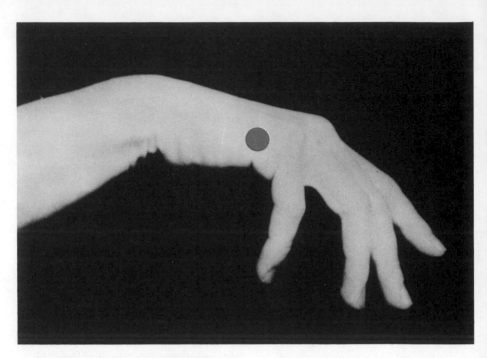

2. For headache on the nape of the neck and back of the head, the effective point is on the little finger side on the hand. Half bend your hand, and you will notice the "head line" crease; your finger extends into it, and you will be able to feel the bone known as the fifth metacarpal. You will feel slight pain when you press on this spot, and you should stimulate at that point. Again, stimulate the right hand side if your pain is on the left side and vice versa.

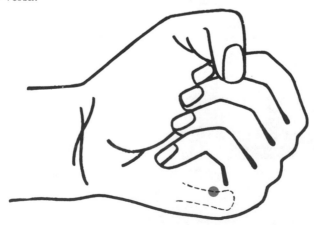

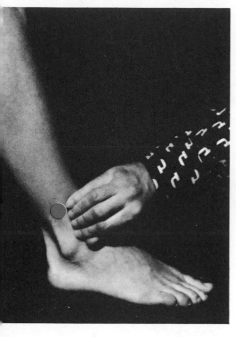

3. For headache in the skull, and generally all over, you can stimulate all the points that apply to 1 and 2, together with the point known as "bladder." This is located at the bottom of the leg, on the outer side, in a small hollow on the front of the long thin bone called the fibula. To find it exactly, with your thumb and fingers together, place the end of your little finger on the protrusion of the ankle bone, and your thumb will indicate the point, as in the diagram.

Press on these two points with your hands crossed.

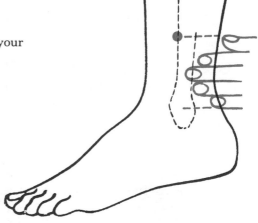

A last word about headaches: the Chinese have always felt that acupuncture is so effective in treating headaches that its failure can only indicate the presence of a brain tumor, or some other serious condition.

To Prevent Colds

The symptoms are familiar enough: you catch a chill, and soon you have watery eyes, a burning sore throat, a runny nose, and you sneeze and feel shivery. You may rush for a hot whisky or brandy — which has never done any good. Alcohol kills germs only if it is applied to them directly with a piece of cotton!

You may say you have the flu, but this is generally inaccurate. Influenza is a major disease that comes in epidemics, and in its most serious form it can kill, in spite of the advances of modern medicine.

Usually what has happened when we think we have the flu is that the lining of our air passages, in other words our respiratory mucous membranes, has been attacked by one of any number of viruses that are going around and give us a cough, a runny nose, and perhaps a fever. What we have is a cold — a condition which the Chinese view as resulting from an unsympathetic energy that invades the body and comes up against the "guard dogs," a select set of the acupuncture meridians. These, according to Chinese theory, are a complex mechanism that we can only mention here in passing, but there are some major points lying along these meridians that should be stimulated. When one feels the onset of a cold, the two main points should be stimulated as soon as possible.

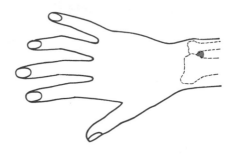

The first point is on the back of the wrist, three finger-widths above the crease.

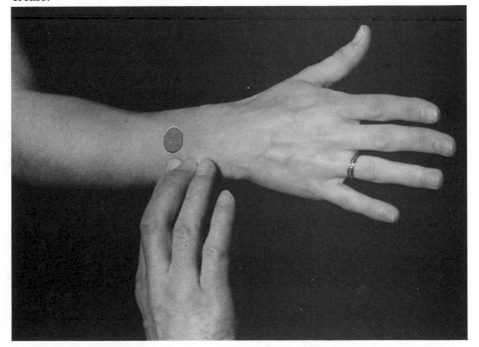

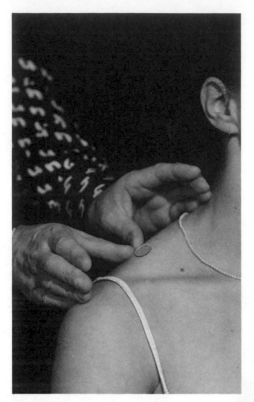

The second point is located on the slope of the shoulder, halfway between the base of the neck and the shoulder tip.

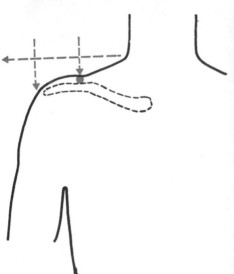

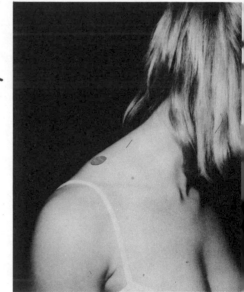

Recovering a Lost Voice

You have a common cold, and suddenly or gradually your voice changes tone, breaks, or just disappears. Or perhaps you've had to shout excessively at a noisy party, or have given a lecture, and your throat has dried up, and you have lost your voice. This is a nuisance in everyday life, but it is disastrous if you use your voice professionally.

How can we explain this curious disappearance of sound? The larynx, the organ that produces the voice, contains a pair of "reeds," which are known technically as the vocal cords. When we speak we cause them to open and close rapidly, and as they move they cause the column of air in the throat to vibrate. By constantly modulating this vibration, they produce the sounds that come out of our mouths.

Two things may go wrong with our vocal cords. First, they may become inert and no longer respond to the signals from the nerves, a condition called laryngeal paralysis. This may be serious, and if the loss of voice does not appear to have an obvious cause, such as a cold or sore throat, it is wise to seek the advice of an ear, nose, and throat specialist so that diagnosis can be made and immediate treatment started.

Second and, fortunately, far more frequently, the cause is either excess use or infection. Inflammation has caused the cords to become swollen so that they cannot move freely and produce proper vibrations. In this instance, acupuncture may be very helpful in relieving the congestion of the larynx, and this allows the sufferer to regain his voice.

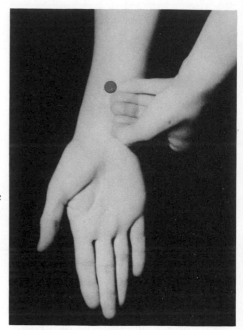

There are two pressure points that are relevant. One is above the wrist. Measure one hand's breadth above the uppermost crease of the wrist, and the point lies on the line that runs up the center of the forearm and divides it in two halves.

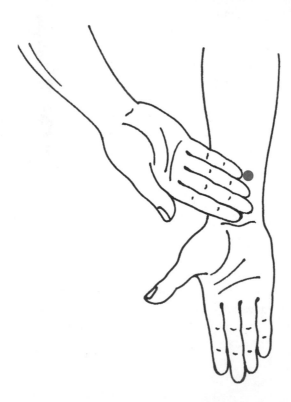

The second is on either side of the little bone called the hyoid, which supports the tongue and its muscles. The position is indicated in the diagram. This point may be massaged gently with the thumb and index finger of the same hand.

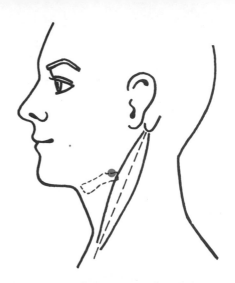

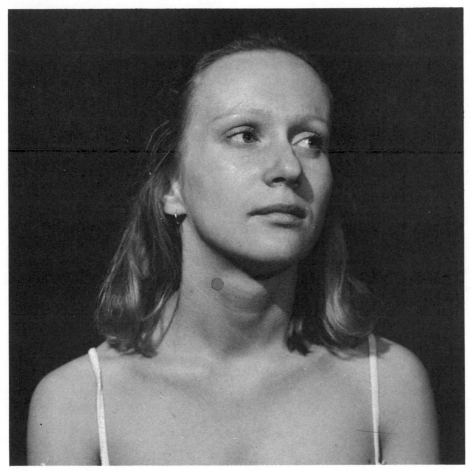

Relief for a Blocked Nose

Unless it is an allergic reaction such as hay fever, this is very much a winter ailment. A stuffed-up nose is often the first sign of any one of a number of virus infections that are common at this time of year: colds, flu, etc.

It may also be caused by a number of chronic infections in the nose and related anatomical cavities. These include infections of the sinuses and the spasmodic catarrh whose springtime form resembles hay fever with its sneezing bouts, continually running nose, and soreness and irritation of the eyes.

The points are the same for all complaints. There are two. One of these is essential and is located in the middle of the forehead above the hairline. If there is no hair, it is even easier to find. Run your finger centrally up the forehead from the bridge of the nose until you reach a small bump, and you'll find the hollow just beyond it. In most people, it is just beyond the hairline. Apply firm pressure to this spot.

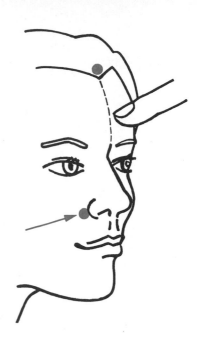

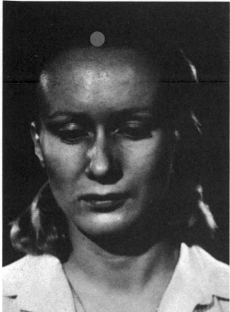

In addition, if one nostril is more congested than the other, there is a point at the bottom corner of the nostril: massage the right side for the right nostril and the left side for the left nostril.

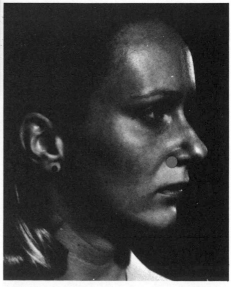

Reducing Sore Throat Pain

A sore throat may be very serious. It can signal the beginning of several other diseases — meningitis, rheumatic fever, or kidney disease — that can have a lasting effect on your life; so unless the sore throat is mild, see your doctor quickly. Meanwhile there is point that will bring relief.

This point is located on the side of the thumb facing the index finger. Draw a line along the base of the nail, and draw a second line at right angles along the side of the nail. The point is at the right angle formed by these two lines. If you have a sore throat on one side only, press the point on this side only. If you have a sore throat all over, press both sides, either alternating or simultaneously.

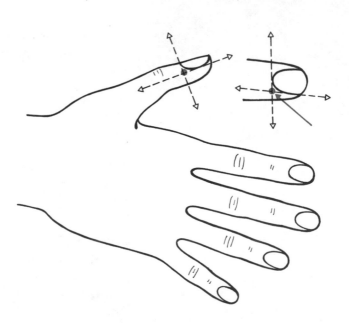

Stopping the Pain of Toothache

Everyone suffers from toothache at some time or another; so it is especially useful to know the effective point for relieving this pain. Luckily it is easily located.

The point is located on the index finger, on the thumb side, at the point of the right angle formed by a horizontal line drawn at the base of the nail and a vertical line drawn at the side of the nail. Use the point on the index finger of the side where the tooth is aching.

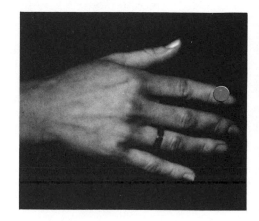

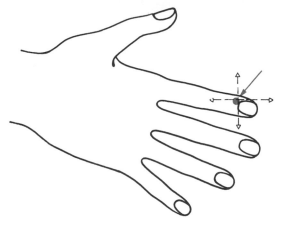

Of course this will not cure decay or an abscess, but it will make the delay until you can see a dentist bearable, and it may even help you undergo treatment without anesthesia. In any case, it is worth a try.

The Skin

Feeling Better after Sunburn or Other First-Degree Burns

Sunburn, unless very severe, is just one example of a first degree burn. The severity of burns is categorized by degrees. In first-degree burns, there is redness of the skin; in second-degree, there are also blisters; a third-degree burn involves complete destruction of the whole thickness of the skin, which becomes insensitive, white, or black if carbonized, and completely dead. Fourth- and fifth-degree burns occur when the muscle or bone is affected.

Only relatively benign burns, like sunburn, may be helped by finger pressure. It is very important to take into account the extent of a burn, for a small second degree burn with a few blisters is much less dangerous than an all-over first-degree sunburn. With widespread first-degree burns, it is wise to see a doctor.

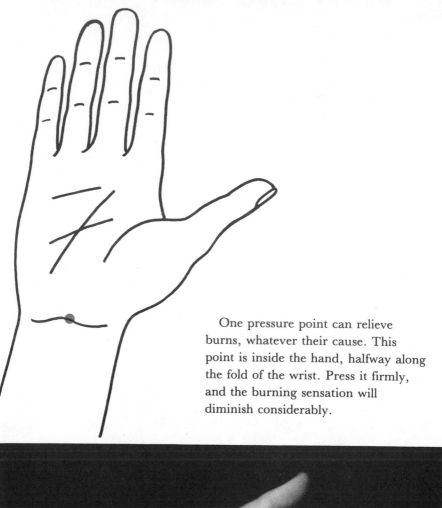

One pressure point can relieve burns, whatever their cause. This point is inside the hand, halfway along the fold of the wrist. Press it firmly, and the burning sensation will diminish considerably.

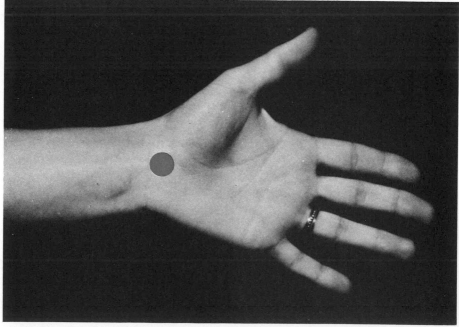

Making Rashes Go Away

There are several sorts of rashes. First, there are those that accompany infectious diseases, such as measles, which are particularly common in childhood. Mostly, apart from chicken pox, these do not itch.

Rashes that do itch, on the other hand, may be of two main sorts. Some are constitutional; they have been with the patient since childhood and often remain throughout life. They demand expert medical care and attention.

Others, however, are fortunately only temporary and are usually linked to an allergy. Allergies are rather mysterious things. A substance that is totally harmless to the vast majority of people causes the patient to break out in a rash. There are several varieties of these rashes, the most common being eczema, with its dry scales and oozing scabs; but there are also hives with their painful, red, velvety swelling that disappears when pressed and that itches dreadfully.

Treatment of an allergy is of course complicated and requires medical advice, but when you break out in a rash from eating strawberries or oysters, for example, it is just as well to be able to relieve the discomfort.

Two points are particularly effective. The first is at the back of the knee, exactly half way along the crease of the joint.

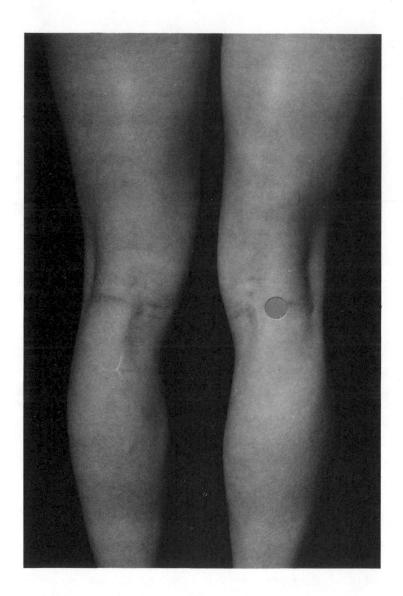

The second is located on either side of the vertrabral column on a level with the third dorsal vertebra. To find it, locate at the base of the nape of the neck a large bony protruberance — this is the spine of the last cervical vertebra. Count three knobs, or spines, below, and you will have reached the third dorsal — our point is on either side of the vertebra, two finger widths along a horizontal line.

To be effective, you need to press vigorously.

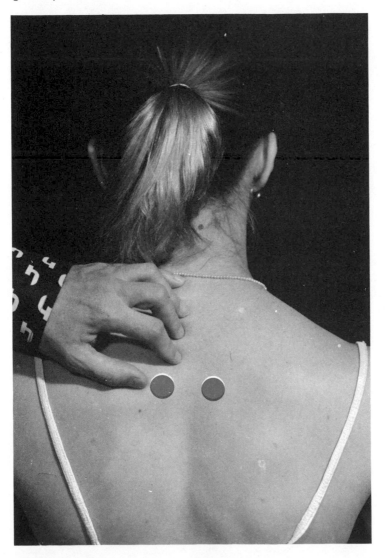

The Chest

To Stop Air Swallowing (Aerophagia)

Sufferers from heartburn are familiar enough with this complaint, and yet there is no straightforward medical definition of it. For a long time the excessive belching of aerophagia was thought to be due to a large amount of air in the stomach, but today we know that when we swallow air it does not reach the stomach. It gets only as far as the esophagus and is then rejected by belching. Frequently with aerophagia we are really talking about a nervous complaint associated with psychosomatic factors.

Belching may also be symptomatic of serious digestive troubles: stomach ulcers, gallstones, and so on, and the stomach distension may also trigger off pain in other areas, in particular, pain in the chest similar to angina.

For these reasons, aerophagia should not be dismissed as unimportant. It is sensible to consult a doctor to find out the specific cause. But in the meantime you will need relief.

For heartburn and a distended stomach, two acupressure points are helpful. The first one is along the inside of the foot. Feel the protrusion of the base of the big toe. Put your little finger on this spot and your other fingers alongside as in the photograph. The tip of the index finger will be resting on the first point as it meets the edge of the bone.

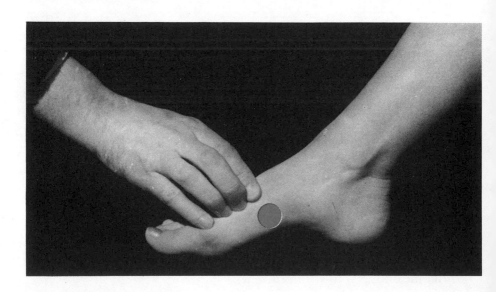

The second point, on the outside edge of the forearm, may be located in the following way: half bending the arm, the point is halfway along the upper edge between the skin creases at the wrist and the elbow.

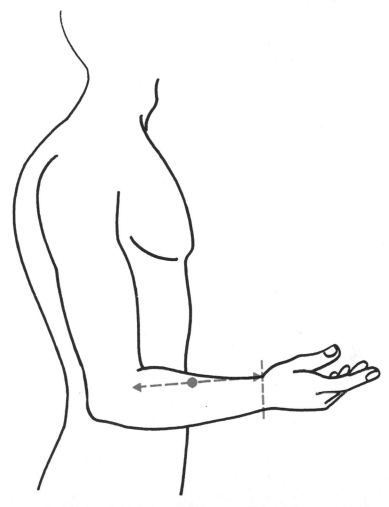

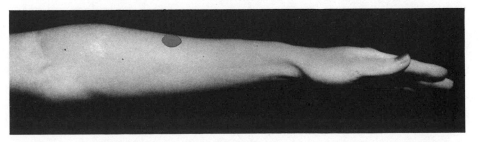

Relief for Breast Pain

Women's breasts are vulnerable areas of the body. They are easily injured and may become painful; they are also susceptible to certain malfunctions and diseases. Women are very aware of the possibility of developing breast cancer; many have learned to conduct self-examination for lumps and do so regularly, especially if their breasts are painful. Pain does not necessarily indicate danger, however. During the menstrual cycle, breasts may swell up and become excessively sensitive, depending on the individual. Mothers who are breast feeding their babies may experience breast pain also, and inflammation of the nipples and the small cysts are a fairly common symptom of breast pain at the time of the menopause.

Of course, if there is something abnormal in the breast you must consult a doctor without delay, but in the meantime there is no harm in relieving your discomfort.

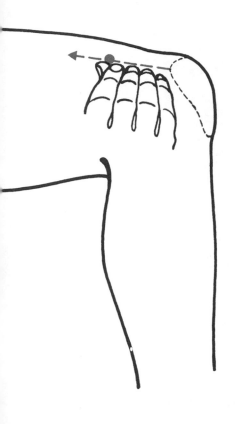

There are two points that provide relief. The first is on the thigh. To find it easily, place your hand above the knee with your little finger just above the outer and upper edge of the knee cap. Your thumb will indicate the effective point.

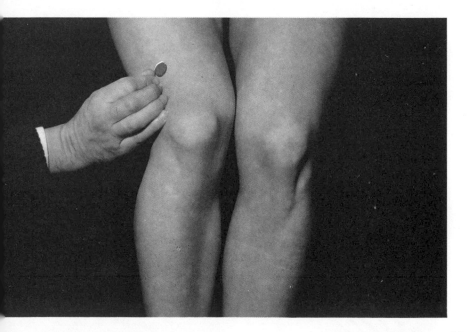

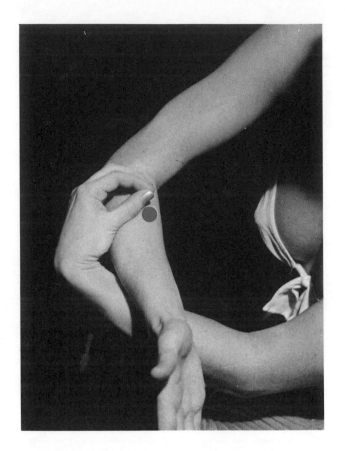

The second point is on the arm; half
bend one arm over the other arm. The
point is three finger-widths below the
fold of your arm, as in the diagram.

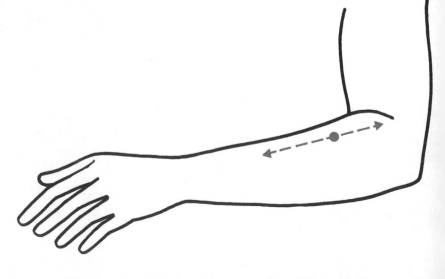

Help for Shortness of Breath

The technical name for this symptom, which may be a sign of serious illness, is dyspnea. Problems of the heart—particularly in older people—the lungs, or the nervous system may be the cause. So if you should develop shortness of breath for no apparent reason, you should see your doctor and perhaps even a heart or chest specialist. But breathlessness may be only a temporary condition arising from a nasty bout of flu or bronchitis, or even emotion. There is also increasing evidence, as a result of research in California and at the London Hospital, that neurological mechanisms and reflexes may be involved, and these, of course, are susceptible to acupuncture.

One disease in particular is characterized by difficulty in breathing, and that is asthma. An asthma attack may be brought on by exposure to a substance such as pollen, to which the person is sensitive, or by an emotional problem. It may cause the patient to wake up at two or three o'clock in the morning, unable to breathe and impelled to sit in front of an open window. Gradually the attacks may become more frequent and develop into a permanent breathing difficulty.

Asthma is an unpleasant illness both for the patient and bystanders, who helplessly witness an attack. There are a number of medicines that may relieve the asthmatic patient of his breathlessness; usually they contain a sort of cortisone, in the form of drops, pills, or aerosol sprays, often combined with drugs to dilate the air passages. But all of these medicines have their disadvantages. First, the asthma victim must always have them with him; and second, all of them have side effects and can be dangerous.

So it is useful to know a method that can bring rapid relief to the breathless sufferer, who must be assisted by someone since the points are located on the back.

63

There are bilateral pressure points located on the back of either side of the spine and two finger widths away from the center, at the level of the third dorsal vertebra. To find this vertebra, the patient should sit down and lower his head. You will notice a projection at the base of his neck, which is the projection of the last cervical vertebra. Going down the back, count three more protrusions, and you will have reached the level of the third dorsal. The points are two finger-widths to the left and right of the spine. The points need to be pressed energetically for a considerable time. Gradually the breathlessness and wheezing will ease and the difficulty disappear, but if the attack is very severe, medical help should be obtained as soon as possible.

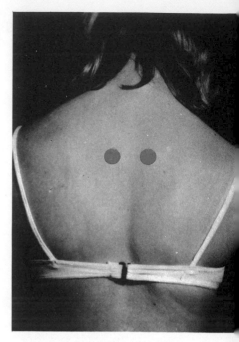

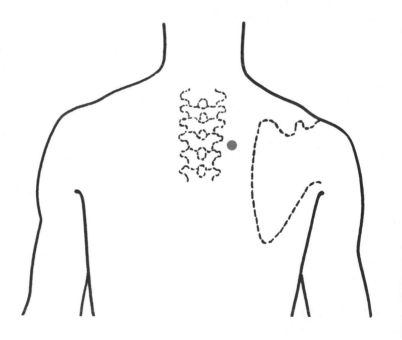

Relieving Chest Pain

Pain in the chest may originate in the organs inside it — the heart and the lungs — or in the chest wall — the muscles, nerves, and ribs. If pain appears without any obvious reason, such as injury, it is wise to take it seriously to start with, and you should arrange to see your doctor as the trouble may be serious, especially if the onset is sudden. Chest pains may be a sign of coronary thrombosis (heart attack), angina (in which case they come on after exertion), or pulmonary embolus (clot on the lung).

However, pains in the chest usually spring from very minor causes, and often the severity of the pain is out of all proportion to the seriousness of the cause. One type of pain that we all have experienced is the "stitch." Another is intercostal neuralgia, which may originate near the vertebra. The chest is also the most frequent site for the eruption of an infectious and very painful viral disease that has the medical name of *herpes zoster*, but is commonly called shingles.

There is a point that will provide relief.

The point is in the middle of the back of the forearm, exactly halfway between the elbow and the wrist. Press it strongly. Using acupuncture in this point, Chinese surgeons have removed parts of the lung without any other form of anesthesia.

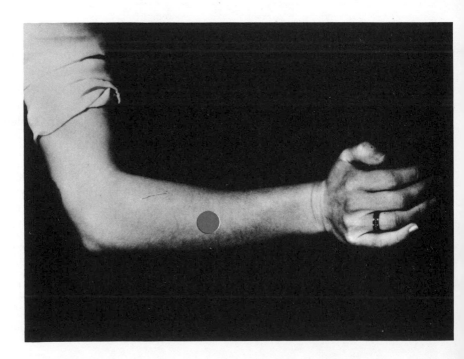

Stopping Palpitations

Are you aware of the heart's astonishing electrical machinery, with its own power station and distribution network that stimulates the cardiac muscle to contract regularly? This power station, known medically as the "pacemaker," normally discharges an electrical signal into the heart about seventy times a minute, and it adapts instantaneously to the needs of the body, depending on whether it is at rest, walking, running, etc. So complex a machine may, of course, go wrong from time to time; the power station may accelerate or slow down, conditions known to doctors as tachycardia or bradycardia; or it can cause an irregular beat, which is called an extra-systole.

The recognition, diagnosis, interpretation, and treatment of these anomalies require detailed cardiographic investigation, and, fortunately, changes in the heartbeat are not often serious. As a rule the complaint is recognized by the patient himself, who feels a sensation of an irregularity — a sudden beat and a pause or a fluttering sensation in the chest. For a few moments there is a feeling of anxiety; the palpitations may be repeated. They may continue for hours and may become a permanent disability. Even if occasional, they can be extremely unpleasant; so it is helpful to try to obtain relief from them as soon as possible.

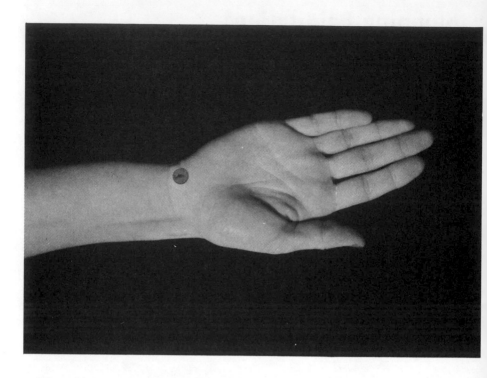

There is one point that is very effective. It is on the inside of the wrist, on the little finger side, at the level of the skin fold along the wrist joint.

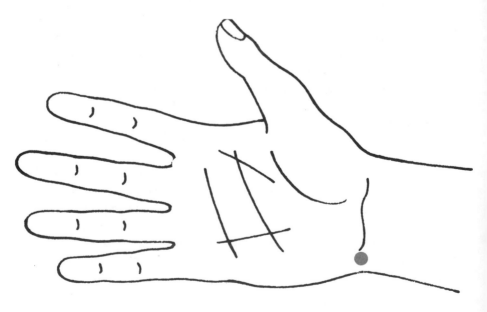

The Abdomen

Stopping Abdominal Pain

Abdominal pain, that is, colic, covers a vast range of complaints:

Intestinal, affecting either the small or large intestine. This is the most frequent site of the pain and may be caused by infection, spasms, cold symptoms, etc.;

Biliary, that is, connected with bile ducts, often caused by a stone;

Ureteric, which may signal a urinary infection or, more commonly, a stone.

In all these cases, and particularly the last two, the pain can be very sudden and excruciating, sometimes even causing the patient to faint.

Relief is as important as diagnosis, not only because you want to alleviate the pain, but also because further pain aggravates the illness. You must try to break the vicious circle, preferably in a way that avoids use of drugs since they sometimes make things worse.

The rapid effect of this pressure point has been the subject of numerous studies. Stimulation has been clearly shown to reduce the rate of intestinal contraction.

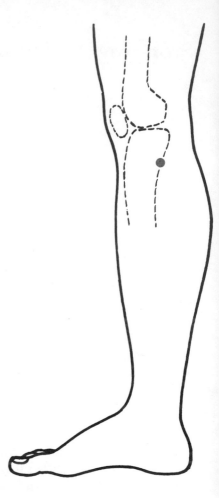

The point is located on the inside of the knee, along the back edge of the tibia. When we follow this edge with the finger, from bottom to top, we find an angle where the edge of the bone suddenly bends inward. The point is at this angle.

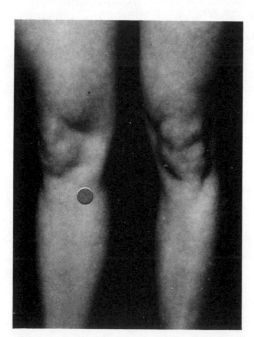

You Ate the Whole Thing

We inaccurately use the term "bilious" to describe such complaints as the distension of the gall bladder or a range of digestive disturbances. We also use it as a polite way to explain the results of overindulgence in food or drink. The pressure point used to relieve such pain is important in the treatment of all liver and biliary complaints.

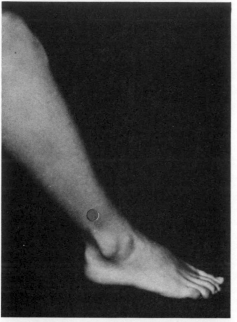

The point is low down on the oute[r]
side of the leg, in a hollow at the fro[nt]
of the long thin bone known as the
fibula.

To find this point, place your han[d]
with your fingers together, on the
outside of your leg, with the little
finger on the most prominent part o[f]
the ankle bone. Your other fingers w[ill]
rest, one above the other, over the
fibula, and your thumb will mark th[e]
spot. Press this point on both legs wi[th]
your hands crossed over: right hand [on]
left leg and left hand on the right leg[.]
After a while you will hear a gurglin[g]
sound in the abdomen. This is the b[owel]
emptying, as radiographic
examinations made during the cours[e]
of the treatment have shown.

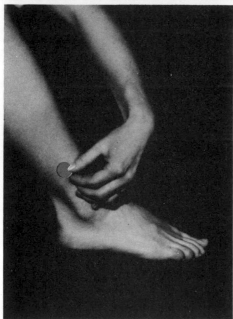

74

Stopping Diarrhea

Diarrhea is very unpleasant. It may be caused by a number of things. It may be serious because it often involves a substantial loss of fluid and essential trace elements, thus endangering the body's well-being. It may be caused by a simple stomach upset or a minor infection, but it can be more serious if it is due to malabsorption or a particularly virulent agent, like food poisoning or dysentery, or caused by a disease that is making a reappearance in tropical countries, even though it was thought to have been almost stamped out—cholera.

Severe diarrhea needs urgent medical attention, but there is a pressure point that is effective in relieving mild cases. I must add that the point is used in China to treat cholera.

The point needs to be located with care. It is a hand's breadth (five finger-widths) below the kneecap on the outside of the leg. And it is halfway between the ridges of the tibia and the fibula.

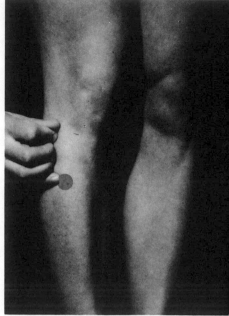

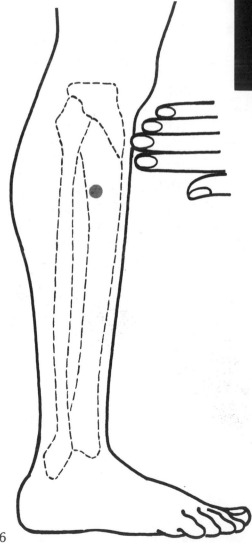

Stopping Hiccups Quickly

We all get hiccups occasionally. They may be embarrassing and if prolonged, an unpleasant nuisance. In rare instances, a person may suffer a dreadfully prolonged attack that may last for days, producing real disability and preventing the sufferer from eating, drinking, and sleeping and bringing him to the brink of a nervous breakdown. Hiccups usually occur when you have swallowed something that has gone down "the wrohg way" or if you have laughed a great deal, perhaps while eating. They are actually caused by sudden contractions, twitches, or spasms of the diaphragm, the thin sheet of muscle that is attached to the lower ribs, and separates the chest from the abdomen. It is one of the muscles of respiration, and normally it rises and falls smoothly. When it twitches, however, it jerks the ribs, the contents of the chest, and the windpipe downward, and that is what is happening when you have hiccups.

Usually the cause of hiccups is quite trivial, but it can sometimes be a symptom of serious nervous disease or chronic kidney failure. Leaving the more serious causes aside, it is desirable to obtain relief quickly from the familiar and unpleasant symptoms of a bout of hiccups. To do this, you will need help, since the pressure points are on the back, near where the diaphragm is attached to the ribs.

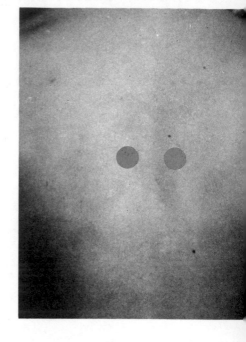

These points are on either side of the spinal cord at a distance of two finger-widths from the midline, on a level with the seventh dorsal vertebra and on the horizontal line joining the lower tips of the shoulder blades, as shown in the diagram.

To apply pressure, the subject should be seated and stripped to the waist.

To Get Rid of Intestinal Worms

You may well ask how stimulation of tiny points on the skin surface can possibly rid the body of those undesirable inhabitants of the lower intestine: worms. Yet, Chinese traditional and practical experience has confirmed that acupuncture is an excellent treatment for this condition. We cannot help asking how this can be possible.

It may be that stimulation triggers off intestinal contractions, which expel the worms. But neither clinical experience nor recordings of intestinal movement have shown this to be the case. We are left thinking that stimulation of the point in some way modifies the environment of the intestine so that life becomes impossible for the parasites. The author of this book has observed that stimulation of this same point has often eradicated cutaneous mycoses (that is, fungal infections of the skin, such as athlete's foot).

So this point appears to arouse the body's defense mechanisms against parasites.

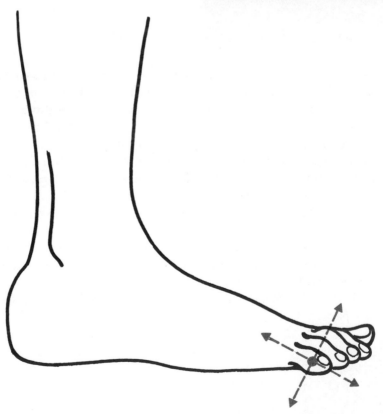

The point is located at the end of the little toe, at the right angle formed by the intersection of two lines, one along the base and the other along the outside of the nail.

To Stop Vomiting

It is beneficial to vomit if you are ridding your body of toxic substances or bad food that may cause trouble once it has passed into the intestines. But vomiting is unpleasant, and in some cases, can be dangerous since it causes loss of fluid and essential mineral salts. In any event, it is just as well to put a stop to the vomiting at the stage where the stomach is empty and yet continues to contract, bringing up only acid, phlegm, and possibly blood.

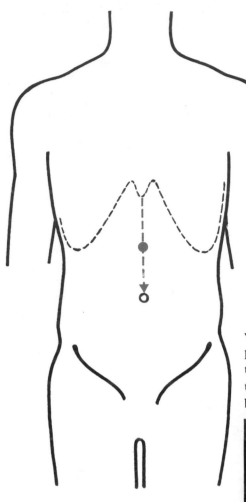

One point is very effective to stop vomiting. It is located on the upper part of the wall of the abdomen, along the meridian line and halfway between the navel and the protrusion at the bottom of the sternum.

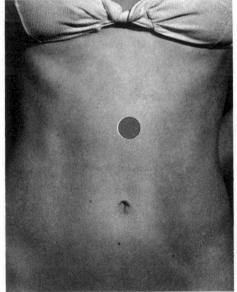

The Anal-Rectal Region

Stopping Anal Discomfort

Anal pains usually make us think of hemorrhoids, and, in fact, this uncomfortable malady is frequently the cause. However, you may be suffering for a number of other reasons: anal fissure, eczema, or an infection such as a boil or an abscess.

Pain from few areas of the body causes so much distress and puts us in so bad a mood. This is as much due to the pain itself as the physiological malfunction that is associated with it since the pain almost inevitably leads to reluctance to open the bowels.

Hemorrhoids, the most frequent reason for anal pain, are varicose veins of the anal region. They are not often a sign of a more serious illness, but if they are causing severe or persistent discomfort it is wise to see a doctor. The cause very often is constipation. The passing of infrequent, dry, and over-large stools tears these veins, causing swelling, bleeding, and blood clots.

These swollen veins then cause the anus to shrink and contract, making the passing of stools even more difficult. Thus a vicious circle is set up in which pain gives rise to muscle spasms in the anus and to further constipation. It is important to break the vicious circle as soon as possible by relieving the constipation and establishing regular bowel habits, but when immediate relief of pain is desired, there is a pressure point that is effective.

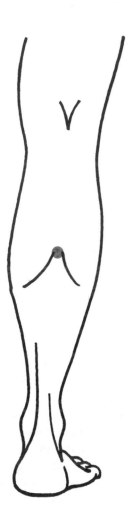

The point is located on the back of the calf, halfway up the leg, just in between the swelling of the two prominent calf muscles.

The point corresponds with and is sometimes used for pain in other areas, but it is particularly beneficial for pain in the region of the anus. It should be pressed bilaterally and deeply, and this is most effective if done using both thumbs.

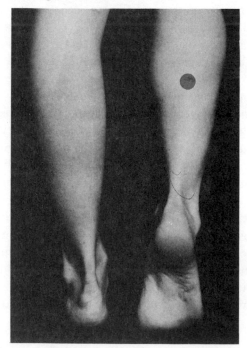

Relieving Constipation

Constipation is a common complaint, a disease of the Western world and of sedentary lifestyles; but it was common in the classical world, too, and laxative remedies have come down to us from the ancient Egyptians.

There is no doubt that lack of exercise together with an unhealthy diet — not drinking enough liquid, not eating enough roughage, green vegetables, bran, and so on — aggravate the problem.

Unfortunately, many sufferers from constipation resort to taking laxatives in the form of pills and medicines, and this merely adds evil to evil. The intestine gradually becomes irritated and inflamed and constipation gives way to diarrhea, which causes dehydration and loss of essential mineral salts; or it may become habituated to the laxative, and larger and larger doses will then be required. Thus further complications arise due to laxatives, which can lead to chronic complaints and even to serious intestinal diseases. Obviously, any natural method that will restore regular bowel movement without traumatizing the body is to be welcomed. Finger pressure is helpful, with one point that is very easy to stimulate.

This point is located at the inside corner of the nail of the big toe, as shown in the diagram.

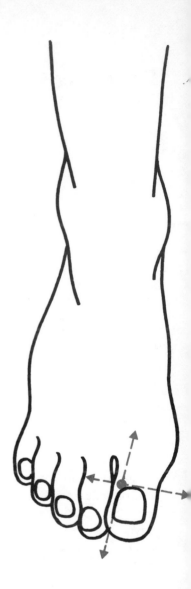

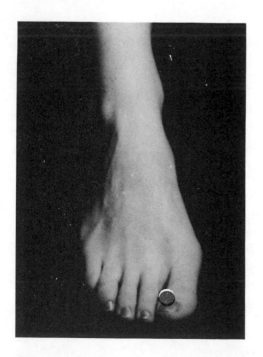

The Shoulders, Arms, and Hands

Taking the Pain out of Tennis Elbow

The elbow is an exposed and awkward joint, which often gets knocked about. It is also often misused, particularly in sports like tennis and golf.

What actually happens in these sports? Sometimes when a swing hasn't quite worked, the forearm goes too far and becomes strained. The pain may be felt anywhere in the elbow, but it is usually on the outside at the lower end of the upper joint bone, the humerus, or "funny bone."

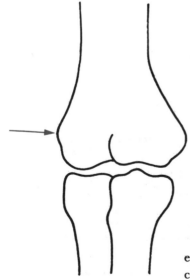

This part of the bone is called the epicondyle and is attached to a whole complex of muscles, tendons, and ligaments.

When one of these ligaments becomes torn or inflamed, we have what is known as "tennis elbow." For a sedentary person, this may be no more than a nuisance, but for a professional sportsman it can be disastrous. So it is helpful to know the point that can often bring immediate relief and avoid chronic complications.

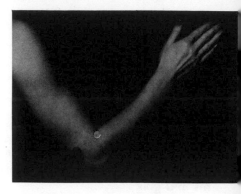

This point is very easy to find. It is at the outer end of the inside fold of the elbow when the arm is bent at a right angle.

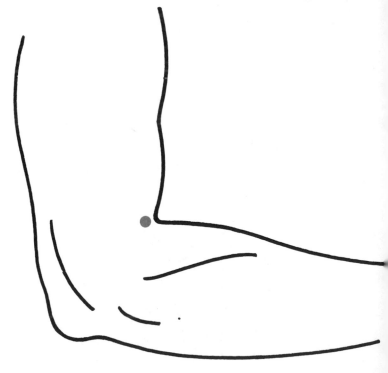

Stimulation of this point may usefully be accompanied by active movements and can be done during or after physiotherapy.

There is no need for complicated equipment. You can find all that you need to exercise your arm in your home: a key in a keyhole or a lock will do.

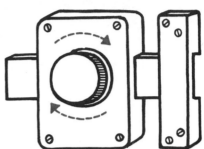

Move your arm slightly back and forth while massaging the point firmly. This will alleviate pain and stiffness.

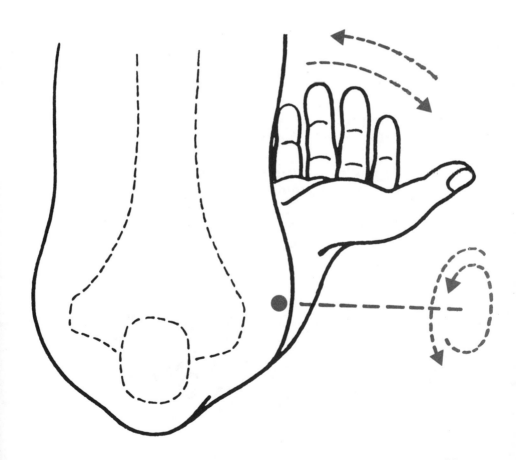

Dealing with Painful Fingers

Fingers are particularly prone to injury. They may be knocked, banged, or strained, or they may be cut, develop infections, or become inflamed.

In elderly people, we often see thumbs become painfully deformed by the development of arthritic conditions.

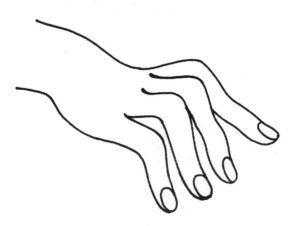

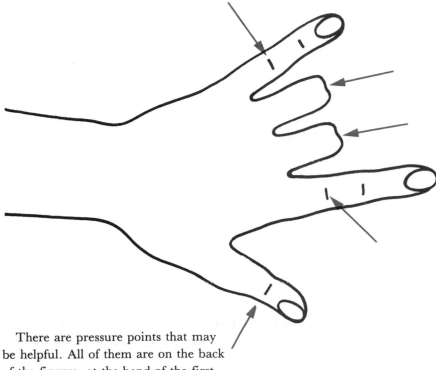

There are pressure points that may
be helpful. All of them are on the back
of the fingers, at the bend of the first
joint.

Stimulate the point on the affected
finger. If all of the fingers are affected,
Chinese tradition dictates the following
order of treatment: first the ring
finger, then the thumb, the middle
finger, the index, and finally the little
finger.

Controlling Shoulder Pain

The shoulder joint often becomes painful. Sometimes the pain is a result of a direct blow, but more often the pain appears spontaneously, and the most serious effect is that it restricts the range of movement of the shoulder and arm, making everyday gestures difficult — fastening a bra, putting on a shirt or jacket, or driving a car, for example. At the very worst, we may suffer from a "frozen" shoulder, which makes any movement almost impossible. This condition may last for a few days or for several months or years. Actually, the joint itself is rarely diseased. The affected parts are the damaged and inflamed ligaments, muscles, tendons, and nerves that surround it.

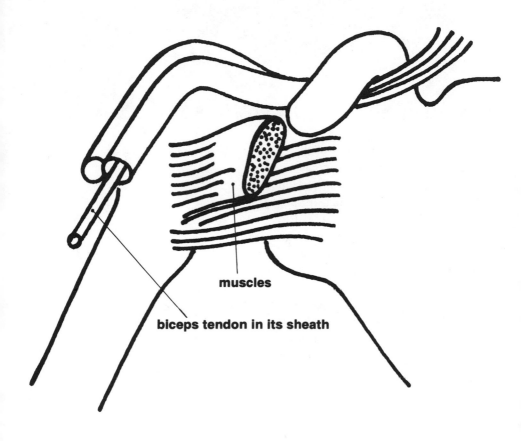

muscles

biceps tendon in its sheath

Medical methods of treatment include cortisone injections in the shoulder region and active and passive physiotherapy, including exercise and swimming. But, once again, there is a point that can quickly relieve pain and prevent the condition from worsening.

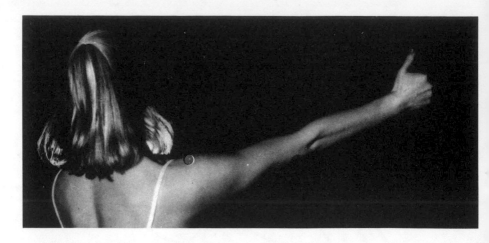

This point is in front of the shoulder, and there is an easy way of finding it. Hold the arm horizontally, with the thumb pointing upward. You'll find a small hollow just in front of the shoulder, and the point is there.

You can also use it during physiotherapy and rehabilitation. It will make your exercises easier.

You may also find a number of painful points around the shoulder by pressing. These will vary from one patient to another. Massage them when the need occurs.

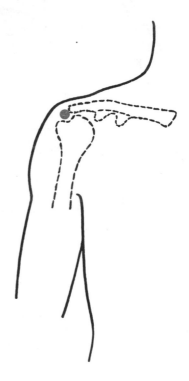

Helping an Aching Wrist or Hand

It is virtually impossible to separate aches in the wrist from aches in the hand. There is a whole network of bones, tendons, and muscles that links the two, as shown in the diagram below.

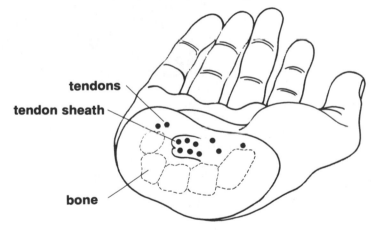

Sometimes a swelling, not always painful, appears on the back of the hand or the wrist; this is a synovial cyst. The synovial membrane that lines the joints between the different bones in the wrist and also lubricates the tendons, herniates through the ligaments and forms a small swelling under the skin. It is filled with a thick viscous fluid, like molasses. This happens after a violent movement has damaged the ligament, often in tennis players, or when straining with a screwdriver; such damage may also occur after frequently repeated movements as in basket making and weaving.

Also, sometimes the ligamentous band across the front of the wrist, which holds the tendons in place, becomes inflamed or shrinks and compresses the nerves that run underneath it. This will produce a neuralgic pain in the wrist or the hand, and signs of swelling may appear around the wrist or the palm.

For all wrist and hand pains, two points are particularly helpful.

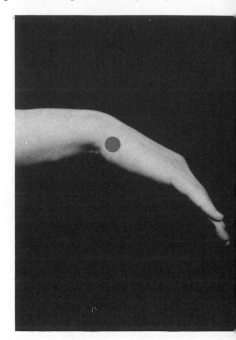

The first is on the little finger side of the hand, a little beyond the wrist, on the second fold that forms when the hand is bent forward as shown in the photo and explained in the diagram.

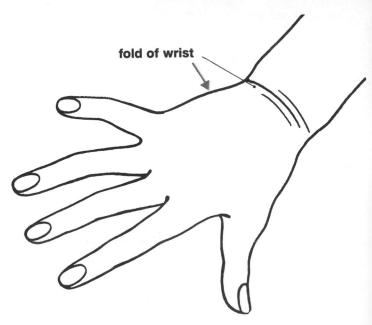

fold of wrist

The second point is located on the back of the wrist, three finger-widths above the fold, just where the two bones of the forearm, the radius and the ulna, meet. This point is very easy to find and feel.

These are the two points to stimulate to relieve a pain in the wrist or hand. They may be used either successively or simultaneously, for as long as is necessary to produce relief.

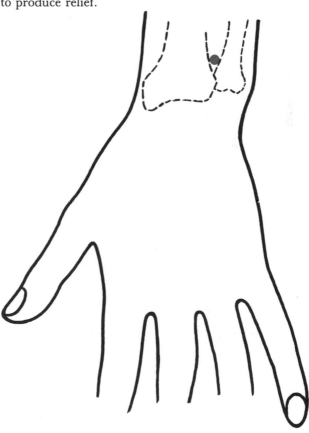

The Hips, Legs, and Feet

Relief for Pain in the Foot and Toes

Our poor feet suffer throughout the year. They may be cramped inside ill-fitting shoes or perched up and distorted by excessively high heels or platform soles. After ten years of such treatment, the feet become deformed, with toes crowded one over the other, fallen arches, and corns and bunions. Walking becomes a torture, and those who suffer the most may seek relief by a surgical operation. The Chinese have been faced with this problem for a long time; their tradition forced the young girls to have their feet bound tightly to keep them small. Inevitably this was painful, and an effective point has been used for a long time to bring relief.

This point is on the foot, exactly at the base of the second toe. Stimulate it forcefully to soothe the pain.

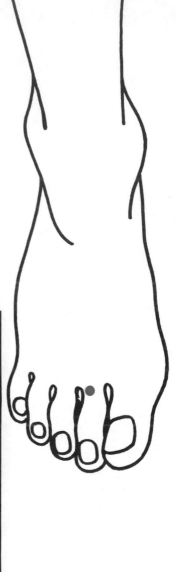

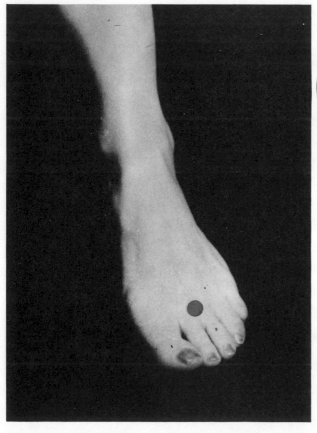

Relief for Leg Cramps

Many people are awakened at night by painful muscle cramps, usually in the calf of the leg. There are two sorts of cramps: one is linked to the blood vessels and is vascular; and the other is linked to malfunctioning of muscles and is muscular.

Among vascular cramps, there are those that result from varicose veins, phlebitis, and all the problems of the veins of the lower limbs. Women are particularly affected by these problems.

Muscular cramps often follow excessive physical exercise and occur, for example, in runners, cyclists, and swimmers.

Whatever the cause, there is a point that will bring quick relief from leg cramps.

This point is located on the calf of each leg, right in the middle, halfway around the back and halfway between the bend of the knee and the top of the heel.

More exactly, the point is in the hollow that separates the two large masses of muscle that become prominent when we stand on tiptoe and that are usually the site of the cramp. This is a deep point, for which firm pressure is recommended.

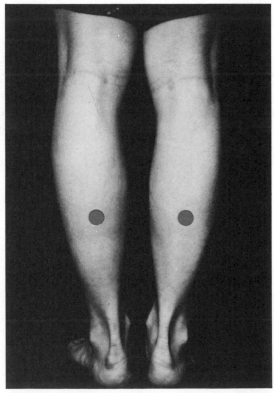

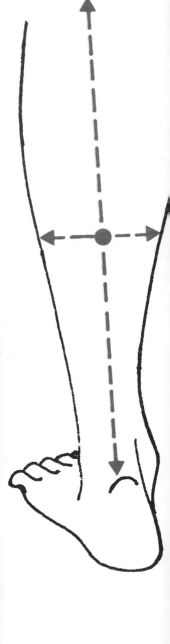

Relief for the Pain of a Twisted Ankle

Twisted ankles can be the result of missing a step or stumbling against the curb, or a similar accident. You should take such an injury seriously; you may have a fracture, and you should be X-rayed. But meanwhile, the ankle is swollen and very painful, and finger pressure can help.

Apply firm pressure to the point located just below the bottom of the ankle bone, either on the inside or the outside, depending on where the swelling is.

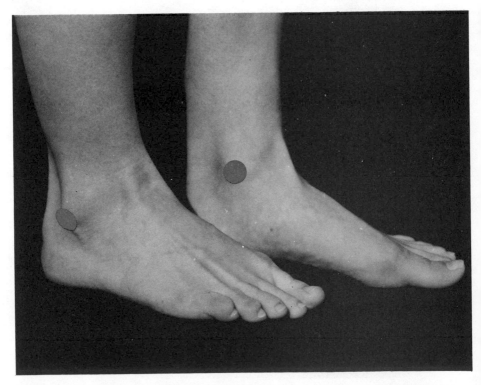

The pain, and even the swelling to some extent, will lessen, and you will be able to walk. Be very careful to keep the finger perpendicular to the skin so that you don't displace anything in case there is a fracture, even a partial one. See your doctor as soon as possible.

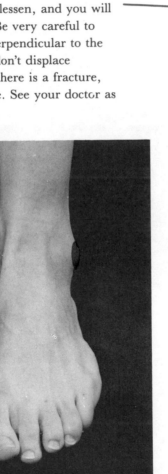

Coping with Pain in the Hip

One thing should be mentioned immediately. An ache in the hip need not arise from a problem in the hip joint itself. It may also be a sign of infection in the abdomen or of trouble in the lower part of the back. This is because the same set of nerves is involved in all these instances. In such cases, the point recommended below will not be of much use, since it is concerned only with conditions in the hip joint itself.

The hip is a deep joint and is generally well-protected by ligaments and muscles, but, as it bears the whole weight of the body, it tends to be affected by osteoarthritis, a slow and dreadfully destructive disease that eventually, after much pain and restriction of movement, finally causes the joint to become fixed in one position.

There have been some brilliant advances in the methods of treating osteoarthritis, and today surgeons can replace the whole hip joint with a metal or plastic one.

However, there is a useful massage point that can relieve pain and help associated treatment, such as exercise, heat, or physiotherapy.

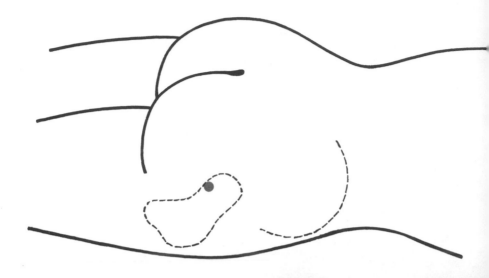

To locate the point, the patient should lie on his healthy side and half bend his affected leg. In this position, the bones—in particular the protrusion of the pelvis and the iliac crest—stand out in relief.

Place your hand along the iliac crest in the following manner: open your hand with the fingers held straight and together, and with your thumb at right angles to the fingers, place the heel of your hand along the crest, with the thumb pointing forward. The tip of your middle finger will then be on the point—in anatomical terms, it is on the bony prominence known as the "greater trochante," as in the diagram, which you can feel under the skin.

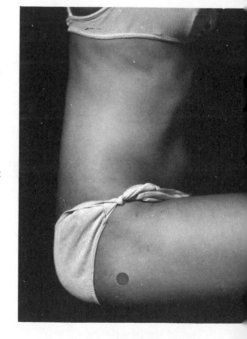

Massage of this point has an effect on all the aches of the lower limb. This is another example of a point that is relevant to more than one complaint (see Sciatica).

Stopping Pain in the Knee

The knee joint is vulnerable to bumps and infections. It is frequently injured in car and sports accidents and is also highly susceptible to a degenerative change in old age, osteoarthritis, which may become very painful. Getting relief is therefore a frequent problem.

In nature, good and evil often go side by side: thus, although the knee is a relatively exposed joint, unprotected by thick muscle masses, the very fact that it is just under the skin makes it very easy to examine and to treat the injured sites.

Besides—and this is valuable for acupuncture as a whole, even when we do not say so directly—a painful point can always be massaged, and this can be as effective as using a specific point, and even more so if combined with it. But there is a specific point for the knee.

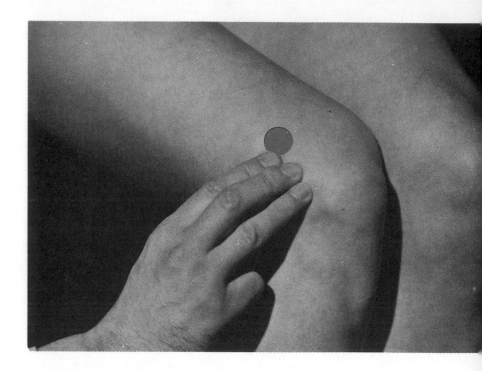

The point corresponds in position with the highest point of the synovial membrane — the little sac that lines the inside of the joint and that, when the joint is injured or inflamed, swells with inflammatory or hemorragic fluid, a synovial effusion.

To locate the point, find the patella, the knee cap, which is the small bone in front of the knee. Our point is three finger-widths above the top of the patella, on the outer side of the thigh, as shown in the illustration.

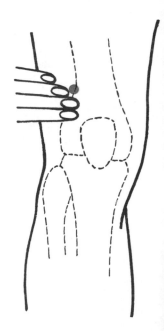

No More Tired Legs

City-dwellers lead a shamefully sedentary existence all week. They sit all day at the office or in the car, then they try to get a week's exercise all on one day. Off they go on Sunday for a walk, a cross country-race, or more violent sports, and it does not take long for them to get tired . . . they can't feel their legs, or rather they can feel them aching only too well!

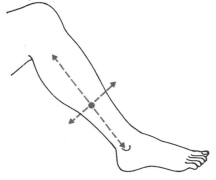

There is a point that is effective in relieving leg fatigue. It is on the outer side of the leg, halfway between the ankle and the knee, just behind the long thin bone known as the fibula.

The point was known in China as the "coolies' point," after the indefatigable men who used to carry heavy loads for days on end without tiring. During World War II, Japanese soldiers, who covered vast distances on foot or by bicycle in the jungle, would burn this point with a lighted cigarette end after every twenty kilometers and carry on again refreshed.

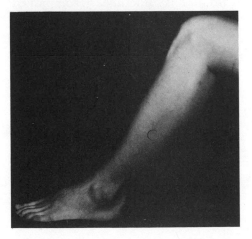

You need not go so far! But if you sit down and press the point for a long time, you will feel that the tiredness in your legs has disappeared.

To Stop Swelling (Edema)

In the majority of cases, it is the lower limbs that are affected by edema. There can be many causes. Some are general; but it is also known that it may be caused by weakness of the heart and kidneys. This is a sign of serious illness, and a doctor should be consulted.

Edema can also be caused by local irritation, such as varicose veins, particularly common in women, in whom it is sometimes accompanied by phlebitis.

There is also lymphatic edema, a condition that is likely to be constitutional rather than local. This is commoner in women and produces tree-trunk-like legs.

Many people suffer from gravitational edema, which appears as swelling behind the ankles and is particularly marked at the end of the day. It occurs in people who have to do a lot of standing or walking, such as salespersons or certain types of factory workers.

In addition to the appropriate treatment and good advice, such as sufficient rest and sleeping with the feet elevated, there is a pressure point that brings relief.

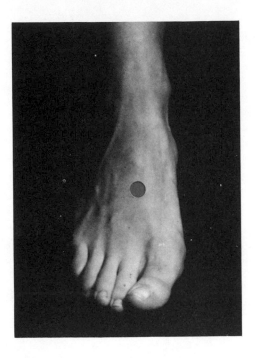

This point is on the foot at the junction of the bones that prolong the big toe and the second toe.

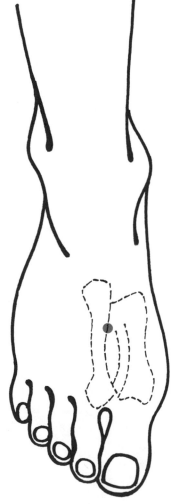

The Back

Relief for Backache

In a society engaged so much in sedentary occupations, the back is inevitably vulnerable. Backache is a familiar enough complaint, brought on for many people because they do not seem to know the correct way to pick up heavy objects. Such lifting should be done by bending the knees and keeping the back straight; the weight is lifted by straightening the knees and is taken by the legs and the shoulders so as to avoid putting a strain on the back. The result of lifting incorrectly, with straight legs and a bent back, is a sudden intense pain.

Even worse may be the chronic suffering of typists, pianists, computer operators, and dentists, for example. This sort of ache is caused by a persistently bad posture, a curving of the back that causes contractions and spasms of the vertebral muscles. Nor should we forget the aching housewife, who bends to make the bed, to wash the dishes, and to do the cleaning and vacuuming day after day!

The back can be affected by many things — from uneven sidewalks to badly worn heels, etc. The vertebral muscles may even be upset by mental disturbance, anguish, and fear, which can cause tense and aching back muscles.

All of this hurts. So it is useful to know a pressure point that will help you relax and prevent persistent pain.

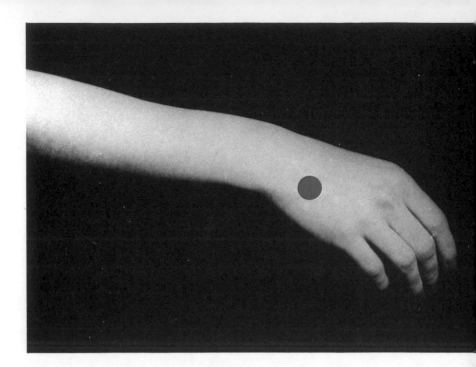

The point is located on the back of the hand at the angle between the bones that prolong the little finger and the ring finger, called the fourth and fifth metacarpious.

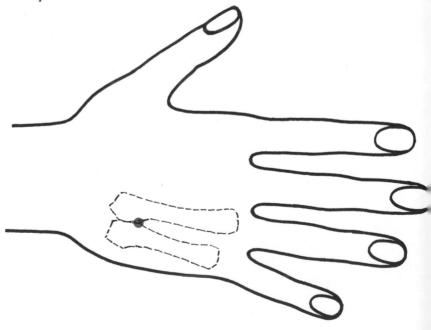

Controlling Lumbago

All of us have suffered from lumbago, or lower backache, at some time or another. It usually occurs after we have overexerted ourselves with the back in an awkward position. Suddenly we feel an excruciating pain — and we are doubled up and incapable of getting up since the very least movement is agonizing. Sometimes the cause is a slipped disc or a displaced vertebra. Whichever it may be, the nerve is caught and pressed on, the muscles contract into spasm, and we feel intense pain. Usually, however, the cause is more trivial — a slight tear in a ligament or muscle, resulting from a sudden twist or strain.

If lumbago isn't treated it may drag on for several days or weeks, improving very slowly until it eventually disappears. Unless you are careful, you may suffer a relapse, if the ligaments, which hold the vertebrae together, do not heal completely you will get these attacks after less and less strenuous exertion. Soon you may have a constant backache, with recrudescences following fatigue and on getting up in the morning. You will have become a chronic sufferer from lumbago.

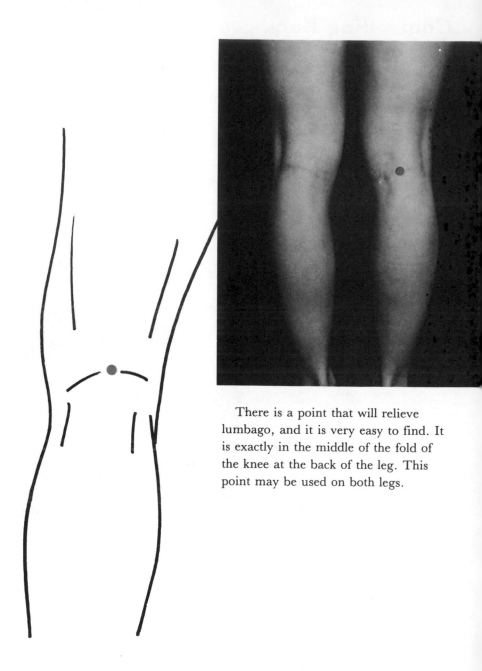

There is a point that will relieve lumbago, and it is very easy to find. It is exactly in the middle of the fold of the knee at the back of the leg. This point may be used on both legs.

Help for Sciatica

This is one of the more painful complaints from which the human being may suffer. As the name suggests, the complaint centers around the sciatic nerve. This nerve begins with several roots at the level of the lumbar vertebrae, and these roots come together into one trunk, which passes down the buttock, the back of the thigh and the leg, and ends right down at the tips of the toes.

We know that sciatica is usually caused by the compression of one or several of these roots — either by the herniation of an intervertebral disc (so-called "slipped disc"), or by displacement or partial dislocation of one vertebra on another, so pinching the origin of the nerve. The pain is felt down the back of the thigh and leg, maybe even to the toes, rather as a message travels along a telegraph line.

Pain is not the only effect since, when the nerve is very much compressed, it stops transmitting completely, and signs of paralysis begin to appear in the leg; this is announced by the onset of the sensation we call "pins and needles," which is an alarm signal for serious complications, and by weakness of the muscles of the leg.

Acute sciatica such as we have just described — which may occur, as with lumbago, and for the same reasons, after a violent effort such as lifting in a bad position — may well improve and even cure itself after a time, but it may also recur and disable the patient without warning from time to time.

Various methods are used to treat sciatica: bedrest; perhaps traction; strong analgesic drugs; injections around the nerve; manipulation to free the compressed nerve root; and, as a last resort, an operation.

Stimulating the appropriate points can bring about considerable relief. These are first the painful points, which you can find along the course of the nerve, and, second, a more specific point, which is equally effective for all pain in the lower limb.

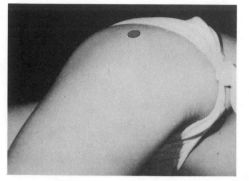

This point is located on the outer side of the buttock, just behind the bulge that constitutes the top of the long thigh bone, the femur, and which is known scientifically as the trochanter.

A good way of finding this point is for the patient to lie down on his healthy side with the affected leg half bent. Place your four fingers along the iliac crest.

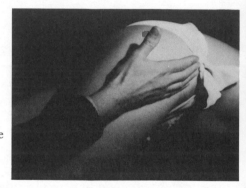

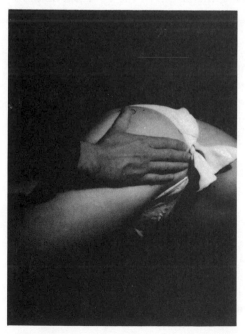

If the thumb is then held at right angles as in the photograph, it will exactly indicate the point.

The Whole Body

Acupuncture and Addiction

The Chinese faced the problem of drug addiction long before the West was even aware of its existence. It is not surprising, then, that they discovered an effective acupuncture point for treatment of addiction to opium and its derivatives; this point is still used successfully in the West as well as in China. What is more, it has been found to be effective also in the treatment of alcohol and tobacco addiction, if used in combination with one or two other select points. Partial or total cure of addiction is, of course, of great importance to us.

The major point for all addiction is the *drug* point. This is located on the side of the skull, exactly in line with the highest point of the ear and three finger-widths above it.

This point is effective for hard or soft drugs: from opium, to LSD, hashish, sleeping pills, etc.

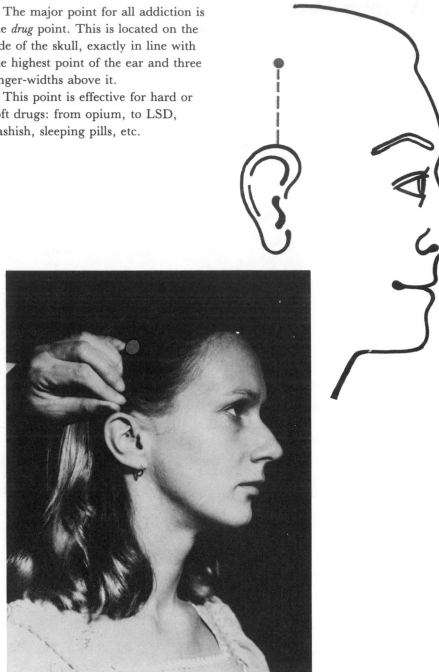

Alcoholism

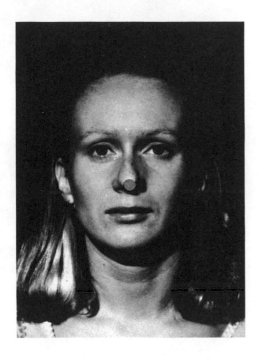

When drunkenness occurs, an additional point should be stimulated. It is exactly at the tip of the nose and is called the *Pi-Tchoun*. Massage here will have a rapidly sobering effect. But be careful: stimulation of this point can cause vomiting. Stand at the patient's side and not right in front of him!

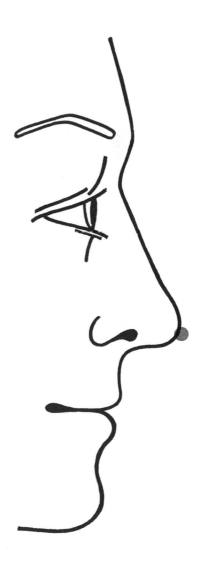

Tobacco

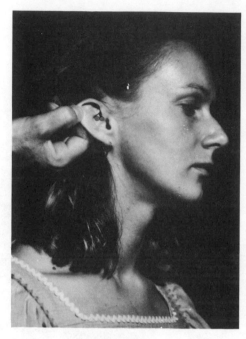

The major *drug* point, as mentioned before, should be stimulated. Two other points on the ear are also effective. One of them is located on the tiny bridge of flesh that forms the "root" of the ear and is called the root or helix.

The second point is just behind the first, almost in the middle of the hole formed by the outer shell of the ear, which is so similar to the inside of a shellfish that it has been called the conch.

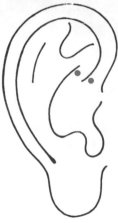

These points occupy a tiny surface area, and it is not easy to find them; but, once located, it is sufficient to press them several times a day and addiction to tobacco will lessen.

The location of these points makes it relevant to mention an interesting extension of classical acupuncture. French researchers — in particular Dr. Nogier — and a number of Chinese have studied an area that until now escaped the attention of traditional investigators. This is the outer part of the ear, and an entire science has arisen out of it — auriculotherapy.

So we can see that the age of discovery in acupuncture is not over, and there may remain other points and useful techniques yet to be revealed.

Help in Getting Over Depression

Depression — this word is heard only too often today. For no obvious reason, over the course of a few days or weeks, a person previously full of energy suddenly loses all interest in life. Work bores him, his family tires him, and entertainment has no appeal. A number of physical effects follow: a suffocating sensation; the feeling of having a lump in his throat; shivering alternating with heavy perspiration; difficulty in sleeping.

As this usually occurs in a very conscientious person, his condition disturbs him; he reacts, cries, rebels, and revolts against the people who surround him. Alternating phases of excitement and despair are characteristic of depression. Little by little, intense fatigue follows the least physical or mental effort. The very idea of moving, of work, of going out appalls the victim. His memory deteriorates, and his family, social, and professional life grinds to a halt.

There are numerous physical and psychological causes of depression. Not the least of these is the pressure of everyday life, the tensions and stresses that affect us all: such abnormalities as air and food pollution, which our bodies must compensate for, long and exhausting journeys, hectic and demanding work; noise; and the frequent interruption of concentration by telephone calls, for example, that seem an inevitable part of modern life.

There is a great temptation for a victim of depression to resort to drugs and tranquillizers, but those who do find they must continually increase the dosage to obtain the same effect. Depression that is severe and prolonged is a serious illness, which requires professional treatment, but even this condition has been improved by use of acupressure.

In such a complex illness, which affects a person in every possible way, there is no single pressure point, but rather a series of zones that can bring relief.

134

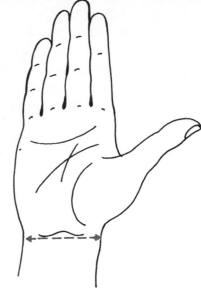

Lie back comfortably, relax, and rub the folds of the wrist that are closest to the palm with the thumb of the other hand, first in one direction and then the other. Then press the hollow of the stomach between the navel and the base of the ribs along the mid-line.

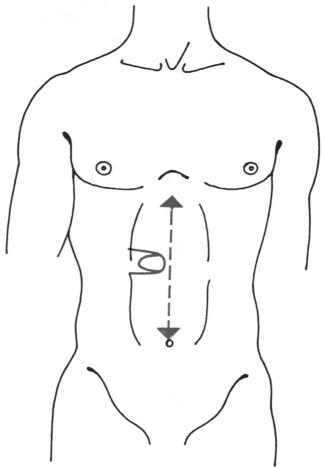

Finally, to complete the session, locate the point at the highest part of the skull, and press it energetically with circular movements. The point will be found along the line joining the ears across the top of the head.

Use this treatment several times a day, and you will gradually notice a sensation of calm that will help you resist depression.

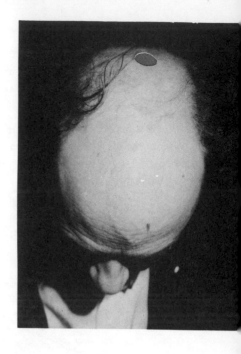

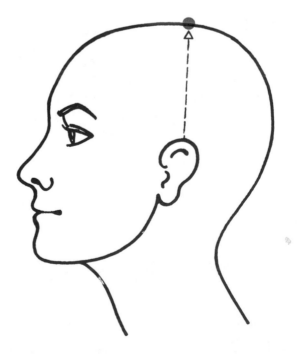

Stopping the Pain of an Injury

In traditional Western therapy, we treat an injury by applying an ointment or cream to the affected area or by taking an aspirin or a similar analgesic.

The Chinese approach to this subject differs from that of the West. In the West, the blow that causes the trauma is seen simply as the cause of the wound, the bruise, the fracture, or whatever it may be. In the Chinese view, the blow has disturbed the defensive energy that covers the entire body like a second skin and flows along the body in certain channels.

They believe that stimulation of a strategic point along one of these channels will improve the patient's condition. It is interesting to note that both the Chinese and Western concepts of shock take into account both mental and physical trauma, even if the shock is psychologically produced, as with bad news.

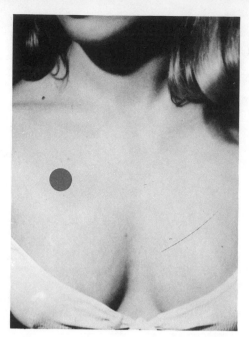

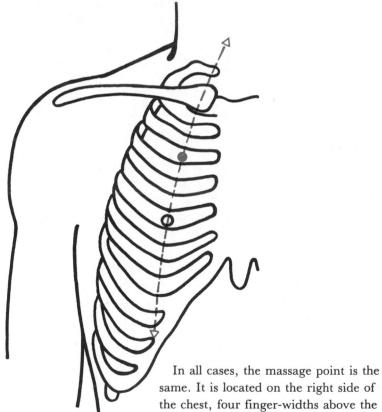

In all cases, the massage point is the same. It is located on the right side of the chest, four finger-widths above the nipple, in the space between the second and third ribs.

Swapping Insomnia for Sleep

You toss and turn in bed—the very bed you've been looking forward to throughout a long and tiring day at work. Your nerves are getting the better of you, and you cannot get to sleep. Or maybe you came home exhausted, slept like a log until two o'clock in the morning, and then you find yourself wide awake. Your mind is full of worries that plague you until the alarm goes off, cruelly announcing that it is time to get up, just when you were beginning to doze off. Insomnia can be serious since continued fatigue and lack of sleep may lead to depression.

So what can you do? Take a sleeping pill? Thousand are bought every day, but it is not the best solution. It has been discovered—only relatively recently—that sleep is not the simple process that we once thought it was. It is a more complex state, involving two levels of unconsciousness that alternate with each other during the course of the night. One level is a deep sleep during which the brain is comparatively inactive; the other level is a paradoxical sleep, during which the brain is very active and the eyeballs move about, so called "Rapid Eye Movement" or REM sleep. It is during REM sleep that you dream, and it has been found—by waking up sleep experiment volunteers—that dreaming is essential for mental health. REM sleep is also the time when your mind resolves the problems that have been troubling you during the day. No sleeping pill can act without disturbing this delicate balance of deep and REM sleep; almost all have been found to produce only deep sleep, leaving the pill-taker with a "hangover" the next morning. The insomnia becomes chronic, and the sufferer has to increase the dosage of sleeping pills, or take stronger drugs with increasingly dangerous side effects, while his health gradually breaks down. So any natural method that can help you to sleep is more than welcome.

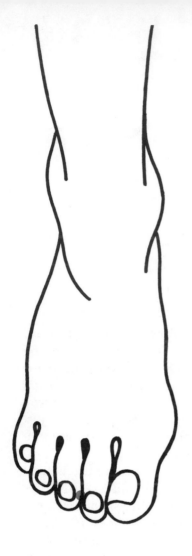

There are two points that will help, and you should massage them slowly. The first one is located at the end of the second toe — the one next to the big toe. The point is at the outer angle of the nail.

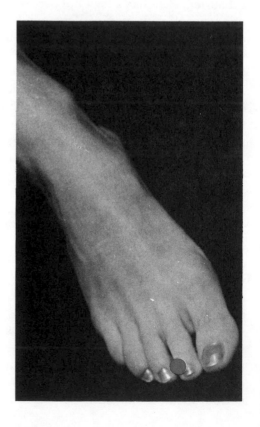

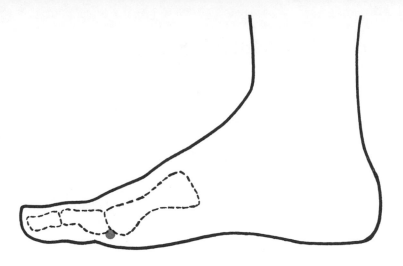

The second point is on the inside
edge of the foot along the side of the
big toe and behind the bony protrusion
at the base of the big toe.

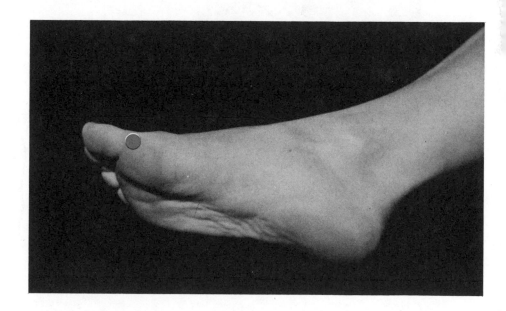

Relieving Motion Sickness

Motion sickness can occur whatever the method of transport — train, car, plane, bus, or boat. It starts with a giddy feeling, then nausea and cold sweats develop, and finally there is vomiting. Sometimes you may be on the point of fainting, and this prevents you from eating as you normally would. Motion sickness can ruin your journey, and people who are prone to it get to a point where they are afraid to travel.

In little children, especially, repeated vomiting can cause dangerous dehydration. It is useful, therefore, to know of an effective point to help prevent motion sickness.

The point is located on the abdomen, right in the middle between the navel and the small point at the bottom of the breast bone. It should be stimulated strongly for a long time.

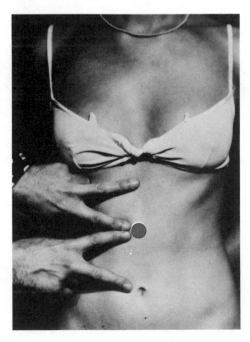 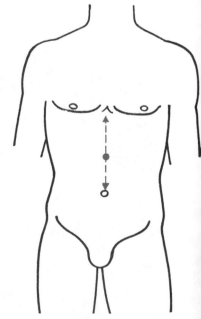

Preventing Stage Fright

The student taking an exam, the singer walking onto the stage, the preacher in his pulpit, or the lecturer in the lecture hall — all may suffer from "nerves" — a dry mouth and throat, a rapid pulse and a throbbing forehead, and difficulty controlling the voice.

Everyone has felt stage fright at one time or another. But for some people it can be a real disability, which can restrict their activities, inhibit their development, and prevent them from fulfilling their ambitions. So it is well worth knowing an effective point that can overcome its effects.

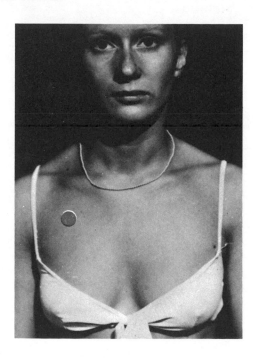 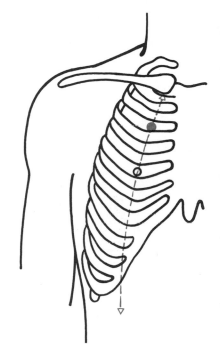

The point, which is also effective for mental and physical shocks or frights, may be stimulated through the clothing. It is high on the right side of the chest, four finger-widths above the right nipple, in the second intercostal space along the mammary meridian. Stimulate it forcefully, and you will calm down and feel relaxed.

Sexuality

Acupuncture and Sexuality

In the West, research into sexuality, for so long a taboo subject, started only relatively recently. According to Freud, of course, our early sexual development is fundamental to the formation of our personality and our adult behavior.

For the Chinese, however, sexual energy is part of our general human energy, which, together with food and the air we breathe, is essential for building and maintaining our vital strength. Maintaining sexual energy is, for the Chinese, not just an agreeable pastime; it is also viewed as being a pressing need for the general health of the body.

A Cure for Impotence

Many factors are thought to contribute to impotence. There may be a physical cause, such as genital abnormality or a serious infection. But today impotence seems to be more often due to the strain and fatigue caused by modern city life or to psychological problems that will have to be traced back to a forgotten episode that may have occurred in childhood or adolescence. Impotence in middle-aged, professional men is a well recognized condition and may be taken as a sign of the extent to which they are preoccupied with their occupations and have time for nothing else. A good relaxing holiday is often a remarkable cure.

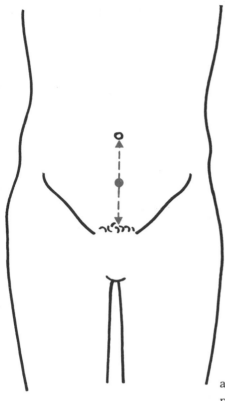

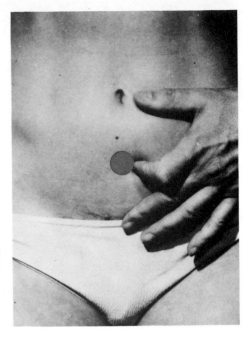

For a speedier and less expensive approach to the problem, there are two points that are very effective. The first is on the abdomen, exactly halfway between the naval and the pubic bone.

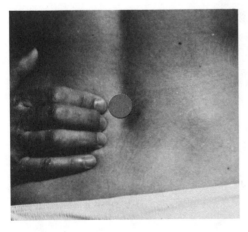

The second is on the back, on the vertebral column, four finger-widths above the large bone known as the sacrum.

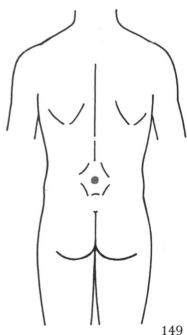

To Treat Frigidity and Infertility

For the Chinese, frigidity, the inability to feel sexually aroused and satisfied, is synonymous with sterility and is thought to affect a woman's ability to conceive.

There are two points. The first is on the inside of the leg. Find the upper end of the tibia, near the knee. Moving your hand down the side, you will feel a bend, and the point is three finger-widths below this, as in the diagram.

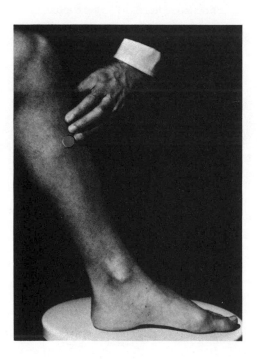

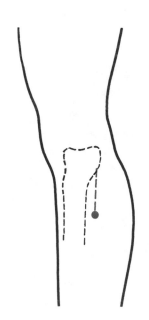

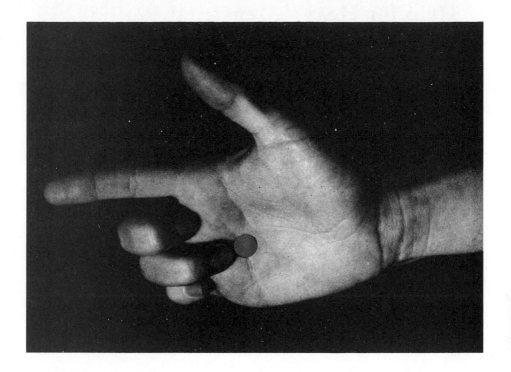

The second point, in the hollow of the hand, is easy to find. It is on the palm, where the finger bends on to the head line.

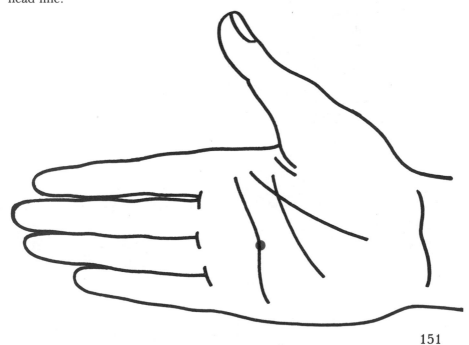

Help for Heavy Menstrual Periods

You may bleed between periods (metrorrhagia) or have periods that are too long or too heavy (menorrhagia). Although many women seem to put up with these complaints remarkably well, excessive or irregular bleeding should have medical attention to avoid complications.

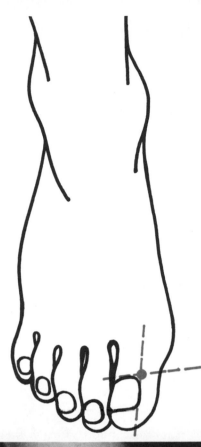

For regulating menstrual flow, there is an effective pressure point on the foot, located in the right angle formed by a line drawn across the base of the big toenail and another drawn along the outer side of the nail, as shown in the diagram.

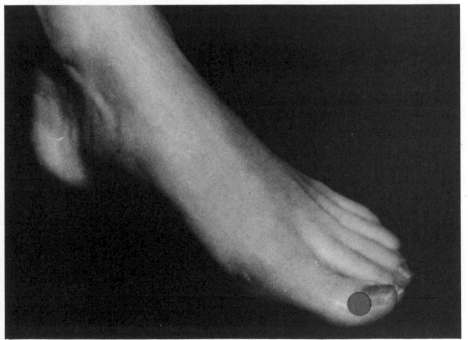

Stopping Menstrual Cramps

Most women suffer varying degrees of discomfort during their periods, whether merely a nagging ache or a violent pain that may even be so agonizing and acute as to cause fainting. Although this is a temporary disability, it occurs regularly and predictably and is awaited with resignation or dread, depending on the severity of the symptoms. The discomforts of menstruation, together with the accompanying psychological disturbances, often have social and professional consequences. Research has shown that women are more likely to be involved in domestic mishaps and even in more serious accidents, around the time of their period.

For the student who has an "off day" and fails an exam, or for any woman who feels so indisposed as to miss a day from work or to cancel her engagements, painful periods are no joke. We need a means of providing fast relief, and there is one point that is very effective for all gynecological upsets.

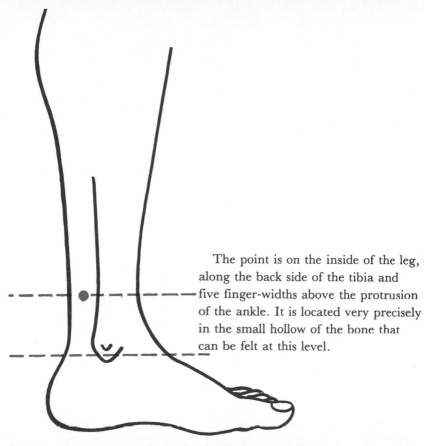

The point is on the inside of the leg, along the back side of the tibia and five finger-widths above the protrusion of the ankle. It is located very precisely in the small hollow of the bone that can be felt at this level.

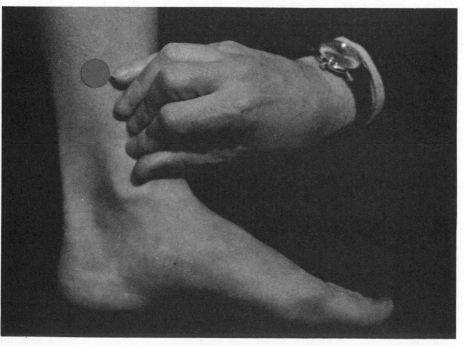

The Scientific Explanation

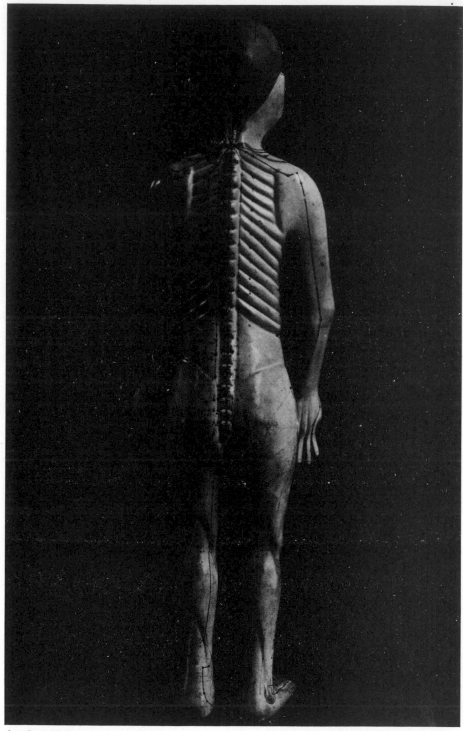

Japanese medicine: acupuncture doll (seen from the back)

Are there scientific proofs of how acupuncture works? This question is frequently asked by patients and doubting doctors. Defenders of the method have little difficulty in producing an impressive and often surprising list of therapeutic successes. But therapeutic successes are not regarded by doctors as indisputable proof since it can be argued that these results might be only the fruit of the imagination, or that the very fact of the acupuncturist's presence sets up a dependence relationship that persuades the patient of the good effects the treatment is having. In other words, they argue that acupuncture is merely a placebo.

Ever since acupuncture appeared in the West, interested doctors have sought to find scientific proof of its method of action (by scientific proof, which is a Western concept, we mean that which is obtained under controlled laboratory conditions).

There are now such proofs of the effect of acupuncture on four systems of the body: on blood composition; on the functioning of the heart; on respiration; and on the digestive system.

It has been shown that stimulation of certain acupuncture points causes the blood to become enriched: a considerable increase in the number of red blood corpuscles appears two or three minutes after stimulation.

Electrocardiogram readings on patients who have disturbed heart rhythms show a marked improvement after acupuncture. The heartbeat becomes more regular both in quantity and in quality.

Respiratory function has been analyzed using spirometers, which register the working of the lungs, and a marked improvement has been observed, particularly in asthmatic patients, whose bronchial spasms die down gradually under the action of the acupuncture needles.

The most spectacular results have been obtained in France recently during observations of the digestive system. The working of the digestive organs has been recorded electronically, using electrodes similar to those of an electrocardiograph but placed on the patient's abdomen. Using these, the movements of the stomach and the intestines, called peristalsis, have been recorded. When peristalsis has been excessive — which may become very painful — the application of acupuncture needles to the front of the abdomen has brought about a considerable reduction of activity and a general calming of the system.

All this is evidence that acupuncture works, but it does not explain how or why it works.

Although the medical profession in the West is prepared to use certain methods of treatment that have been found to work in spite of the fact that they do not know the reason for their effectiveness — this particularly applies to certain forms of psychiatric treatment — there is a surprising resistance to the use of acupuncture, which has also been shown to work, but for which, until very recently, it has not been possible to provide a scientific explanation. For this reason, it has been very important to investigate the actual mechanism by which acupuncture works on the body.

Recent research in the Western world — in France, Scotland, Canada, and the United States in particular — has produced a number of discoveries that throw light on the way in which acupuncture, and even finger pressure, may produce an effect.

The Mechanism of Action at Skin Level

Let us start with evidence for the action at skin level. How can we register proof that something particular is happening at the points and meridians of acupuncture? For a long time, it has been observed that stimulation of the points along the meridian network results in a different pain sensitivity from that of neighboring tissues.

Recently, experiments have been made with electric currents administered at the acupuncture points, and it has been observed that sensation is felt more intensely by the subject at these points than in adjacent areas, to the extent that the pain was felt to be unbearable in the former while scarcely any at all was felt in the latter.

For a very long time investigators tried unsuccessfully to find the reason for this. First, they tried examining samples of skin, either from cadavers or volunteers, from immediately over the acupuncture point. They put the samples under a microscope to see if there was anything different there — a nerve ending, a particular little corpuscle. They found nothing. It is true that this research was done some time ago with an optical microscope. Experiments have not been done with an electronic microscope, which might reveal something.

However, doctors have spent years recording electrical currents and resistance at the acupuncture points and meridian lines and comparing these with other parts of the skin; but until recently all such results were open to the criticism that the smallest amount of pressure on the skin will alter resistance, and this, of course, includes the pressure exerted by the recording electrodes themselves.

In New York, however, Dr. Becker and his associates have been using teflon, rather than metal, electrodes; these have the advantage that they exert minimal pressure, thus eliminating error as far as possible. Using this new technique, it has been found that electrical resistance and conductivity are different if measured between acupuncture points and meridians and other areas of the skin.

Electrical conductivity is greatest at the points and decreases sharply in surrounding areas. There is an oval area around each point away from which conductivity decreases gradually. Thus there is direct evidence of the existence of the points themselves.

Similarly, it has been shown that conductivity is greater along the meridian lines than elsewhere. Becker and his colleagues placed two electrodes a few centimeters apart along one of the meridians and set up a parallel pair one centimeter away from them. Electrical current passed far more readily along the meridian line than along its parallel. Consequently, *it is certain that there are specific electrical properties at the points and along the meridians that are different from those of the surrounding tissues.*

The results of this research have been the starting point of new hypotheses, which are currently being investigated. The general theory of Becker and his colleagues is that there is a nervous system in the skin that developed earlier and is more primitive than the central nervous system, probably a remnant from an earlier embryonic stage. The human embryo, as it develops, passes through a stage when it is similar to an amphibian or a fish with gills. At this stage, before the definitive central nervous system has formed, a primitive nervous network appears, which persists at skin level. It is a system concerned with the defense and growth of the skin, and it comes into action throughout a person's life; for example, to bring about the healing of injuries to the skin. It is suggested that acupuncture acts through this system and that the system acts as a transmission network, with the meridian lines functioning as cables, and the nuclei, where the information is at a maximum, acting as centers that amplify and reinforce the amount of energy in the system.

It is astonishing to see how this modern American theory ties in exactly with the Chinese concept of the *acupuncture points as energy junctions that relay and reinforce energy along the meridian lines and that organize the passage of this energy through the skin toward the organs and the central nervous system.*

There is an extraordinary similarity between these two theories, which are four thousand years apart, and we shall note this similarity again when we come to consider the mode of action of acupuncture on the spinal cord and the central nervous system.

The Mechanism of Action
at Spinal Cord Level

To understand the theory of how acupuncture influences the sensation of pain in the spinal cord, it is first necessary to know something about the anatomy and physiology of pain and to learn a little medical terminology. The classical conception of the transmission of pain was very simple. The earlier researchers knew that there were nerve terminals in the skin and the various organs, and they thought that all types of nerve fibers could transmit all types of sensation, whether cold, warmth, touch, or pain. These nerve fibers terminate in the back part of the spinal cord, in the area known as the posterior horn. From here the pain message ascends to the brain, and it is in the brain that the message is identified as being painful; it becomes "pain."

It is now known that there are two types of nerves concerned with the transmission of pain sensations. The first group, known as A-delta fibers, are relatively thick and insulated; the second group, the C-fibers, are much finer and are not insulated. Impulses are transmitted much more quickly in the A-delta fibers than in the C-fibers, with the result that when we hurt ourselves we feel first, almost instantaneously, a sharp pain sensation and then, after a second or so, a duller but more prolonged pain. This is because the sensation of being transmitted to the brain at two speeds through the two types of nerve fiber, and the pain is experienced as two separate sensations a little while apart. By inserting electrodes into the nerve fibers, it has been possible to record the electrical signals passing along them and to show the difference in speed with which the signals are transmitted. All these nerves terminate, as we have mentioned, in the posterior horn of the spinal cord, in a region called the *substantia gelatinosa* because of its jelly-like appearance. In this region, they make contact with cells that are connected, through the long nerve tracts that run up the spinal cord, with the brain. In the *substantia gelatinosa* region also, it has long been known that there are large numbers of small nerve cells, but until recently it did not seem that they had any purpose.

Pain perception varies greatly, not only between different people but in the same person from time to time, depending on all sorts of circumstances, such as distraction of attention from the pain itself by something of greater interest. We have all heard of the sportsman who has finished the game in spite of injury and has been oblivious to the pain of a deep cut or fracture until it started to hurt when the game came to an end and his attention was no longer diverted from it. An explanation of this and other variations in pain sensation was proposed in 1965 by two doctors, one British and the other American, Professors Wall and Melzack. As a result of their research into the small cells in the *substantia gelatinosa,* they concluded that these cells acted as a "pain gate," switching on and off the transmission of impulses from the pain nerves into the cells of the spinal cord. This has become known as the *gate theory* of pain. Wall and Melzack suggest that the pain perception mechanism is influenced partly by signals coming down from the spinal cord from the brain and controlling the small switching cells and partly by nerve impulses reaching the *substantia gelatinosa* through a different group of nerve fibers coming mainly from the skin and the muscles, called the A-beta fibers. These A-beta fibers are quite thick and insulated, and they end in the region of the small switching cells in the *substantia gelatinosa*. They carry the signals for such sensations as touch, rubbing, vibration, pressure, and temperature, and if the signals are very frequent and intense they cause, to a greater or lesser extent, the switching off of the pain signals. Conversely, if there is not much activity in the A-beta fibers, the pain fibers are switched on. It is not suggested, of course, that a physical gate exists. The word "gate" is used metaphorically, in the same way as it is used in electronics, to signify the switching on and off of a circuit by means of electrical signals.

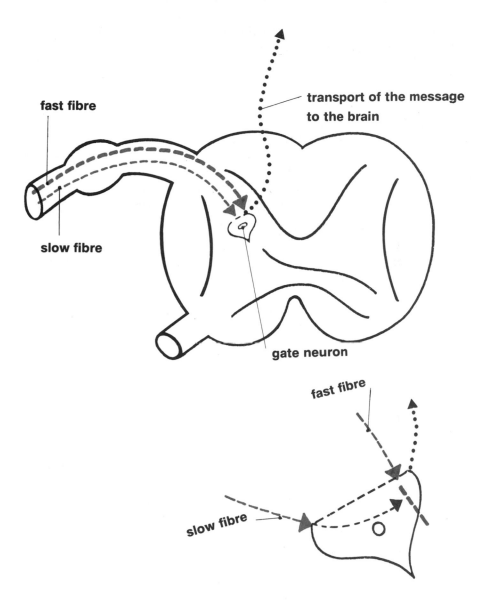

fast fibre

transport of the message
to the brain

slow fibre

gate neuron

fast fibre

slow fibre

This gate theory explains how it is possible for pain to be dis-regarded, either by a conscious decision in the brain or because the brain's attention is so intensely concentrated on something else that it sends switching-off signals down the spinal cord. It also explains how pain sensations can be affected by things happening at skin level. Rubbing the skin when one is hurt, or warming it, sends signals along the

A-beta fibers that switch off some or all of the pain corrections in the *substantia gelatinosa.*

It is beginning to be shown that some of the A-beta fibers terminate in the skin at the principal acupuncture points; so stimulation of one of these points will trigger off a continuous signal to the spinal cord, thus "shutting the gate" and blocking the passage of painful sensations to the brain.

This, in part, explains how surgical operations can be performed using acupuncture instead of conventional anesthesia. According to Chinese tradition, by stimulating the appropriate point before, during, and after the operation, painful sensations are blocked, and the surgeon can operate in a tranquil atmosphere, with all the advantages for him and for the patient.

What can be done in surgery may also be useful in treating medical conditions, including those that have been described in the preceding pages of this book.

The Mechanism of Action at Brain Level

One of the most recent and exciting discoveries about the way in which the brain works has been shown to be closely related to the effects of acupuncture, and it is a strange and surprising coincidence that the research was originally concerned with something apparently quite different. Scientists were trying to discover how morphine, a drug known and used to relieve pain for the last three or four thousand years, worked in the brain. Using a new and powerful research technique, they made an unexpected discovery.

The Structure of the Brain

Like the rest of the body, the brain is made up of cells, which are the building blocks of living matter. In the brain there are several varieties of cells, some of which have the purpose of providing support, defense, and nutrition for the brain; but we are interested here only in the real nerve cells—the neurones. Here, again, we must use some medical terminology. As with all cells, the neurones are composed of a nucleus and a body—which we call protoplasm. But certain of the neurones are different and distinctive in that they have one long prolongation, a filament called an axon, and a number of much shorter filaments, called dendrites, sticking out from them.

To get an idea of what one of these neurones is like, imagine a floor lamp with hairs growing out of the top of the lamp. The pole represents the axon, the bulb part of the lamp is the cell itself, and the hairs represent the dendrites.

Now the axons are actually the nerve fibers that we spoke about in the last section. They may be very long indeed. In the sciatic nerve, which is the longest nerve in the body, they are up to three feet long, depending on how tall the person is. The actual neurones, the cells, of the sciatic nerve, are in the spinal cord, but the axons extend as far as the tips of the toes and transmit messages to and from them. Messages, or nervous impulses, as they are called, pass up and down the axons like an electric current, by a method known as depolarization. When the impulse reaches the neurone, it has to be passed on to the next cell in the chain for transmission up the spinal cord and to the brain. This is the function of the short, fine filaments, the dendrites. They make contact with the surface of the adjacent cell, and under the microscope they look a bit like the tentacles of an octopus attached to its prey.

The method of transmission of the impulse from one cell to the next is quite different from the way it passes up the axon. We have seen that in the axon it flows up like an electric current. From one cell to the next, however, it is transmitted by means of a chemical substance produced in the first neurone and passed by means of the dendrites to the second. A very complicated mechanism is involved in the production of this chemical messenger by the first neurone and in the means by which it is released and sent off to make contact with the second neurone. When it arrives there, it is identified by and attaches itself to a special site on the cell surface, rather as a boat enters a harbor and ties up at its place of anchorage. The effect of this chemical reaching its special site has been compared with the effect of inserting and turning a key in a lock; if it is the correct key, the door is opened. If it is the wrong key, the lock jams. In the neurone, when the "right key" is turned in the lock, the receiving cell is stimulated, and the message passed onward, again electronically; and the chemical messenger, its task completed, is rapidly destroyed.

Until recently, only one chemical messenger was known to exist. Then modern methods of analysis revealed another, and then more. At the present time, a number of different chemical messengers, so-called "transmitters," have been found—adrenalin, serotonin, dopamine, gamma aminobutyric acid—some of these stimulate the brain, others depress its functions, and there is now growing evidence that they may be concerned in the causation of mental illness if they are present in abnormal quantities.

The consequences of these discoveries are staggering. The nerve cells are really glands, capable of secreting chemical substances and often sending them off some distance; and not all cells secrete the same substance. This varies, depending on the region of the brain and its special functions — as one might say, depending on the message, so the "messenger" changes.

Natural Drugs

After these very exciting discoveries, scientists moved on to thinking that this junction between neurones might not only be a zone of great activity but also an area of great sensitivity, susceptible to injury or poisoning. As we have said, inserting the wrong key jams the lock, and a number of drugs are known to act like the wrong key at these junctions; for example, the aerosol insecticides and curare.

Some researchers then considered the effect of various intoxicating substances, some quite dangerous and not used medicinally as drugs, so-called psychedelic substances; and, with the object of helping addicts, work has been done also to investigate the action of narcotic drugs on the central nervous system — in particular, hard drugs such as opium and its derivative, morphine.

Using radioactive methods, it has been found that morphine is accepted by certain nerve cells in the brain. These neurones have at their surface specific sites to which morphine molecules can attach themselves — once again the notion of anchorage that we mentioned above. When this was first discovered, it caused great excitement among scientists. It was thought to be extraordinary that nature could foresee that a vegetable substance — from a flower, the poppy — would enter into contact with the nervous system to the extent that its arrival was perfectly well prepared for. Then came the flash of inspiration. If such an alien substance was accepted, it must be similar to a natural secretion of the brain itself. As so often today, demonstration followed quickly upon the idea, and within a few months, at Aberdeen University and the University of California at La Jolla, a series of chemical messengers in the brain, chemically very similar to morphine, were discovered. These have been called endorphines, or natural morphines, and they have the same effect as the drug morphine, that is to say, they suppress pain. They appear to work by blocking the transmission of pain impulses from one neurone to another, like the wrong key in the lock.

There have now been discovered a number of these substances, all rather similar chemically, which are known to have a calming, or even a euphoric effect, producing optimism, or even joy, according to their chemical structure and the place of production in the brain, the pituitary gland, or elsewhere.

The Role of Acupuncture

What has all this to do with acupuncture? A Canadian scientist, Professor Pomeranz of Toronto, made the crucial discovery: acupuncture liberated these very endorphines. The idea of looking for this effect came to him — so he tells us — when he saw the way the Chinese use acupuncture before surgery; they stimulate the acupuncture point for at least twenty minutes before starting to operate, and this is the time necessary for the formation of the chemical substance, the endorphine. Pomeranz gives these proofs:

(1) Cerebro-spinal fluid, the fluid that bathes the brain and spinal cord, taken from a subject anesthetized by acupuncture transmits this sedative effect to another who is not acupunctured. This is evidence that there is a chemical substance present in the cerebro-spinal fluid of a subject treated with acupuncture which has effects that may be transmitted by injection.

(3) Using electrodes attached to the brain of an animal, Pomeranz registered the reactions of the neurones to pain. The reactions are signaled by a certain number of "blips" on the trace. These blips, signifying the transmission of painful impulses, diminish and then stop completely when the acupuncture point is stimulated, even though pain is still being provoked.

(3) Finally, Pomeranz used a chemical substance that blocks the action of morphine and of endorphine in the brain. This is a morphine antidote, naloxone, a wrong key, which, attaching itself to the morphine site on the surface of the neurones, prevents morphine from producing its usual action. Naloxone also has the effect of preventing acupuncture from relieving pain, and it also reverses the pain relief already produced by acupuncture if it is injected afterward. This is virtually proof that acupuncture acts by stimulating the production of endorphines.

But Pomeranz goes further. He deduces from this that prolonged action demands similarly prolonged stimulation, from twenty minutes to an hour, and, whichever the method of stimulation — injection, electricity, or simple pressure — the result obtained has an identical effect on the pain. Isn't this a justification for the methods described in this book?

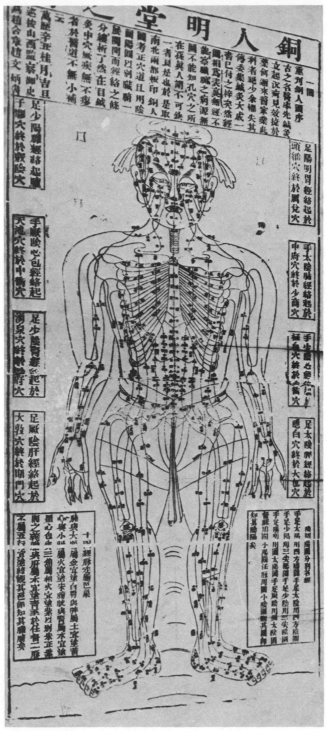

Chinese medicine acupuncture diagram

173

Conclusion

You are now ready to provide relief for yourself if you are suffering from one of over fifty common disabilities described in this book.

As we have said more than once, we are talking about temporary relief; for full diagnosis and treatment you should consult your doctor. But at least you can abate the pain and prevent it from getting worse. And perhaps your observations, of which we would always be glad to learn, can help advance a branch of medicine that has strong connections with the past and holds rich promise for the future.

We will be more than satisfied if we have aroused your curiosity and enabled you to relieve some troublesome complaints.

Statuette showing the affected part of the patient's body.
Women would send these to their doctors.
(Photo: Roger Viollet)

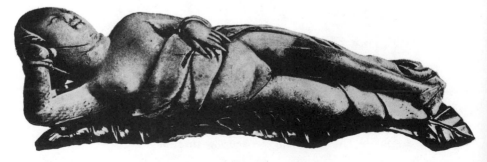

Index

Menstrual cycle:
  breast pain in, 60
  cramps, 154–55
  heavy periods, 152–53
Metrorrhagia, 152–53
Middle ear, infection of, 21
Migraine headache, 27
Morphine, 167, 169
  antidote to, 172
Motion sickness, 142
Mucous membranes, irritation of, 36
Muscular cramps, in leg, 107

Narcotics, addiction to, 129–30
Nausea, 142
Nervous system, diseases of, 63, 77
Neuralgia:
  facial, 26
  intercostal, 65
Nose, blocked, 42–43

Opium, addiction to, 129–30
Osteoarthritis:
  in hip, 111
  in knee, 113
Otitis, 21
Overindulgence, 73–74

Palpitations, heart, 67–68
Paralysis of leg, 125
Parasites, intestinal, 79–80
Peristalsis, painful, 160
Phlebitis, 107, 116–17
Pulmonary embolus, 65

Rashes, 51–53
Renal colic, 29
Rheumatic fever, 44

Sciatic nerve, 125, 168
Sciatica, 125–26
Sexuality, 147–51
Shingles, 65
Shock, 137, 143
Shoulder, painful, 96–98

Sinus infection, 42
Skin, painful, 49–53
Sleeplessness, 139–41
Slipped disc, 123–24, 125
Sore throat, 44
  and loss of voice, 39
Sprained ankle, 109–110
Stage fright, 143
Sterility, 150–51
Stitch, 65
Stomach:
  distended, 57–59
  ulcers, 57
Stones, gall and kidney, 71
Stuffy nose, 42–43
Sunburn, 49–50
Swelling of legs, 116–17
Synovial cyst, 99

Tachycardia, 67
Tennis elbow, 91–93
Throat, sore, 44
  loss of voice, 39–40
Thumbs, arthritic, 94–95
Tired legs, 115
Tobacco, addiction to, 129–30, 132–33
Toe, painful, 105–06
Toothache, 45

Ulcers, stomach, 57
Unconsciousness, 29 30
Ureteric colic, 71
Urinary infections, 71

Varicose veins, 107, 116–17
  hemorrhoids, 85
Vascular cramps, of leg, 107
Vertebra, displaced, 123–24, 125
Vertigo, 29–30
Voice, loss of, 39–41
Vomiting, 81–82
  motion sickness, 142

Worms, intestinal, 79–80
Wounds, 137–38
Wrist, painful, 99–101